RACING THE CLOCK

ALSO BY BERND HEINRICH

Bumblebee Economics (1979)

Insect Thermoregulation (1981)

In a Patch of Fireweed: A Biologist's Life in the Field (1984)

One Man's Owl (1987)

Ravens in Winter (1989)

*The Hot-Blooded Insects: Strategies and
Mechanisms of Thermoregulation* (1993)

A Year in the Maine Woods (1994)

The Thermal Warriors: Strategies of Insect Survival (1996)

The Trees in My Forest (1997)

*Mind of the Raven: Investigations and
Adventures with Wolf-Birds* (1999)

*Racing the Antelope: What Animals Can Teach
Us About Running and Life* (2001)

Winter World: The Ingenuity of Animal Survival (2003)

The Geese of Beaver Bog (2004)

*The Snoring Bird: My Family's Journey Through
a Century of Biology* (2007)

Summer World: A Season of Bounty (2009)

*The Nesting Season: Cuckoos, Cuckolds, and
the Invention of Monogamy* (2010)

Life Everlasting: The Animal Way of Death (2012)

The Homing Instinct: Meaning and Mystery in Animal Migration (2014)

One Wild Bird at a Time: Portraits of Individual Lives (2016)

*The Naturalist's Notebook: An Observation Guide
and 5-Year Calendar-Journal for Tracking Changes
in the Natural World Around You* (2017)

White Feathers: The Nesting Lives of Tree Swallows (2020)

RACING THE CLOCK

RUNNING ACROSS A LIFETIME

BERND HEINRICH

ecco

An Imprint of HarperCollinsPublishers

HarperCollins books may be purchased for educational, business, or sales promotional use. For information, please email the Special Markets Department at SPsales@harpercollins.com.

Ecco® and HarperCollins® are trademarks of HarperCollins Publishers.

FIRST EDITION

Designed by Michelle Crowe

Library of Congress Cataloging-in-Publication Data has been applied for.

ISBN 978-0-06-297327-6

21 22 23 24 25   LSC   10 9 8 7 6 5 4 3 2 1

Tell me and I forget. Teach me and I remember. Involve me and I learn.

—XUNZI

CONTENTS

Preface

LIKE MANY OTHERS, I WRITE IN A DIARY TO KEEP TRACK OF THE passage of time by what is going on in my life. Runners write to see if they're still on course to reach a goal of running a certain distance in a specific time. I'm loaded with a double goal: I had proposed to myself to run a 100k at age eighty and set an age-specific world record doing it, using myself as a guinea pig and then writing a book about it.

I'm mostly a biologist, and observing the nature around me, asking questions, and doing experiments has been my life's work. I'm always on the lookout for suitable subjects. I've experimented on sphinx moths, honeybees, bumblebees, butterflies, syrphid flies, dance flies, giant dung beetles, dragonflies, winter moths, crows, ravens, sapsuckers, iris flowers, American chestnuts, red squirrels, and more, then published my discoveries. The older I have become, the more it has struck me how much all of life has in common. We are all kin. And so I sometimes apply what I learn to us humans and have experimented on myself to test a variety of racing fuels, such as honey, cranberry juice, olive oil, chocolate ice cream, beer, baby food, and yeast rolls, preferably each with multiple trials (excluding an inadvertent one during a twenty-four-hour race on cranberry juice that was sweetened with a chemical other than sugar). Aging is also a trial of one, and I've been at it now for seventy-nine years. I proposed to document my attempt to run that 100k soon after my eightieth birthday, on April 19, 2020.

But right now, I'm sitting on my couch next to the wood-stove in the mountainous, near-endless forest of western Maine, where I've lived continuously for the past ten years and which was my spiritual home for about sixty-five before that. It is snow-ing hard, and the wind is blowing. Glancing at my calendar, I see that I'm already eighty years plus three days old, and also see the 100k race target date and place, April 26 at Lake Waramaug in Connecticut, entered there last November. However, we've been months in lockdown because of the global pandemic. Last week even the Boston Marathon was canceled. Leaving aside COVID-19, I was already out of the running by the end of No-vember, after I chased a deer one afternoon in the first big snow-storm and ended up in the rocky crags of Houghton Ledges, on a mountain adjacent to the cabin where I live, with an ankle in-jury that still precludes serious running. As I am now incapable of even conceiving of running 100k at one stretch, my daily diary is tilted toward what I see nearby in the woods. This morning at 4:46 a.m., still in the dark, I noted, "All is snow-covered. Seems like midwinter. But just now the woodcock, more commonly called the 'timber doodle,' is out there in my clearing in the woods on the snow. He is announcing his presence at dusk and dawn by a repetitive 'peenting' call while perched on the ground, to then perform one after another of his spectacular sky dances, as though nothing had happened despite the snowstorm yester-day and last night. I wonder what else will be up when daylight comes—will the Phoebe, the Hermit thrush, the Winter wren that came back probably too early retreat south, or will their biological clocks not allow them to change from their normal schedule of being here now to sing and to nest?"

Science is a search for authenticity and proof. At least in physics, chemistry, and perhaps astronomy, that is revealed, or presumably achieved, in part by the aid of mathematical formulae, which do not concern time directly (Einstein's famous formula of energy equals mass multiplied by the speed of light squared does so indirectly, since speed is a function of time). But to us, time is an almost universal and viscerally felt component, life is anything but certain, and it is as true as the law of gravity that literally everything in life concerns time. There would not have been any evolution, not even a virus or a cell, without time: no birth, no dying. Time is at the root of our lives, and there are always currents simultaneously pushing and pulling us from various directions whose outcome can be explained by the laws of physics and chemistry.

I am awed by the way trivial incidents, which happen continuously, have profound influences as they ripple down seemingly to the end of time and how each road closed can create a time to reevaluate and open a new one, to reveal other possibilities that could not even have been encountered or thought of before. Every day is a potential disaster or an opportunity.

To paraphrase the poet Robert Frost, I still have many more miles to go and promises to keep. However, my original plan of running a 100k ultramarathon is not going to happen. I'm realizing at age eighty that I no longer feel the fire, the need to do that one specific thing regardless of the circumstances and the consequences. Who knows how long the COVID-19 lockdown will last? It may outlast me. I can now do some other things better than run, and I'll take that.

After seeing the writing on the wall and having been given

more time, since I didn't need to do my daily twenty-mile training run, I reached back in memory, rummaging among a stack
of paper-filled cardboard boxes piled up under the cabin eaves.
They hold jumbles of notes from courses taught, background
material of books written, research done, notebooks and letters,
and lots and lots of running files dating all the way back to my
cross-country days as a junior and senior during my six years at
the Good Will–Hinckley Home Farm and School in Hinckley,
Maine, a school for kids without homes.

One of the boxes was inherited from my parents and recently
passed on to me by my sister. I had not seen it before. It contained all the letters to and from my parents ranging over the
twenty-eight years I had been separated from them, starting at
age twelve at Good Will. In my letters to Papa and Mamusha
(as we called our Polish-German mother), I had complained because my housemother had forbidden me to write in German,
after she had found me doing so. Papa wrote letters that were
first in German and like mine later, in English. They were longer than some of my research papers, and in one he wrote, "I
am sorry and sad you don't like it [there]. There are always such
times in one's life, but later one comes back to one's hobbies;
maybe you should try sports."

Another letter I had written to Mamusha was dated April 9,
1956. I had been there for four years. It was, as were all my letters at that time, written in German, and I started it by telling
her that my knife was now "fixed" (I was mixing languages by
then) and that it had a good point so that I could again throw
it as before. I was then in the "American frontiersman pioneer
in the wilderness" stage of my developmental cycle. I also told
her that the snow had just melted and that many robins, tree
swallows, song sparrows, crows, and even a killdeer were back,

and indirectly that my bees, which I had hived from a bee tree the previous fall, had survived the winter in the hive, because on Thursday I had gone to be near them and got stung on the back of my head. I also wrote, "*Freitag bin ich nicht in die Schule gegangen aber in den Wald*" ("Friday I did not go to school but into the woods") and "*da bin ich in ein* stream *gefallen*" ("there I fell into a stream"—the German would have been *Bach*) that I had tried to jump over. I had then found a dry spot, undressed, and lain naked in the sun and almost fallen asleep. My letter is written in pencil, but in the blue ink in my mother's handwriting at the top of the first page is a curt note saying that a week later "*Bernd weg gelaufen*" ("Bernd ran away"). There was no mention that two days later I arrived back home at the farm. The day after I had run away from school, she noted that I had been taken right back to it. The one-way distance from that "home" to the one I felt was my real one had been a bit more than that of a marathon. It did not exhaust me but instead made me hungrier for the woods. The farm had been planned only as a stopover, to the destination I presumed to be the endless woods about twelve miles beyond (the very same where I have now been living off-grid, off and on for forty years). Living in the woods in a homemade log cabin, living off the land like the pioneers, was something we learned about in school, and it seemed the coolest thing I had learned so far. But at the time I could only dream of it.

By then I had a number of hobbies, including baseball, tennis, swimming, skiing, raising caterpillars, and looking for birds and their nests. Track was not offered by the school, but we did have a gravel pit where I practiced long jumping, and there was a rope hung from a great sugar maple tree where a couple of us boys practiced hand-over-hand climbing and our knife throwing.

I developed my focus on running only in my last two years of high school. Running is among the most intense and universal activities of our species. Its imprint is visible to any biologist in the comparison of our bodies and our minds to those of our closest relatives. Running as a sport was then being offered at school and called "cross-country"; we ran and raced over some of the same woodsy trails I already knew well. But running for me goes back to when I was five years old, reaching back to my parents' struggles and their extraordinary lives and through my finding a home in both biology and in running. Now, with no second 100k record attempt on the horizon, I reach back into memories, letters, contacts, and my career as a biologist and scientist.

A week before my eightieth birthday, I received a letter from a man in Montana who said he had been running his whole life, ever since he was able, which he said was "at two," and he had just turned forty-two and intended to run "as long as I am able to. But," he continued, "I wake up stiff and my morning runs often are of a plodding nature." He had bought my book *Why We Run* years before and, having just read it, thought I might have advice, having at his age set world records. So he was soliciting recommendations from me for running less with a "plodding nature" for someone of "his age." I've been asked the same question, since I was still a youngster at age forty, of guys pulling alongside me on the highway. They ask, "Hey, Ben, you still running?" All I can say is "I hope so." But a time will come when I'm just plodding, due to the unstoppable biological clock. Some things—especially running—get a lot harder for all of us, and they are or become seemingly impossible to many. But are they really? How much does perception derived from habit and experience make it the road not taken?

This book concerns aging, but it doesn't contain advice or recommendations about running. With "old" age approaching, the choices may become ever fewer and farther between, with less time left to make the right ones. Those choices, dictated by the biological clock, can then become less skewed toward achieving a predetermined race result and more focused on taking things as they come and making the best of them. That may sound like a cop-out. But "making the best of it" is being realistic about what we have achieved or can achieve rather than what we think we must or should achieve.

One lesson I have learned is that life is a journey, and too-careful planning of the road ahead can lead to a dead end and frustration. Looking back, I see magic when seemingly devastating setbacks led to unanticipated opportunities that could not be wasted. But some things are inevitable. And what time does to us is one. All life must adjust to its effects. This fact of life is perhaps especially conspicuous in running, which is deeply rooted in the meaning and mechanisms of our biology. There are some things to give up and other things to lean toward. What are they, and what are the differences between them?

1

The Biological Clock

FEW THINGS IN THE WORLD SEEM MORE IMPORTANT THAN time. We all have a physiological clock that influences our lives, yet we scarcely know what time is. Time exists not as a thing or an event in itself but only as something *between* events, and we are all acutely aware of it. Physicists continue to ponder it, and it is biblically enshrined by the famous truism in Ecclesiastes: "To everything there is a season and a reason for every purpose under the heaven; a time to be born and a time to die, a time to plant and a time to uproot, a time to kill and a time to heal, a time to tear down and a time to build."

Our biological clock is hardly precise. Certain of our genes control it, and we see what it does, but we don't yet know how it works. It was perhaps most vividly first demonstrated in bees and flowers by the Austrian beekeeper and biologist Karl von Frisch, who made an amazing discovery in the 1950s proving how honeybees communicate the distance and direction of a profitable food source to their hive mates. I'm awed by the beauty and the elegance of his experiments, so clear and succinct that even a child could understand them, as I did when my father gave me Frisch's thin little book *The Dancing Bees: An Account of the Life and Senses of the Honey Bee* for my sixteenth birthday. He inscribed it with my name and then *"Dem Imker von seinen Vater zu Weinachten* 1956" (The beekeeper from his father for Christmas 1956). Papa thus acknowledged me for something I had already been passionate about for four years. But I'm starting with Frisch here now because of an unanticipated and seldom mentioned secondary discovery of his bee studies, one highlighting the biological clock.

The bee's internal clock runs on an approximately twenty-four-hour schedule. Frisch noticed that while feeding his bees sugar syrup in the field, they came back to search for that food not only at the place where he had provided it but also at the time (to, on average, within fifteen minutes) when he had fed them there previously. But that alone didn't clinch the fact that bees can tell time. More evidence came from the apparent "dances" (which were in fact messages) that he watched closely as he deciphered how they encoded the information indicating the flight direction and distance to a food source. Each dance is a code for a symbolic flight performed on a vertical honeycomb in the darkness of the hive, directing recruits to the distant food source. It indicates to the bees attending it the direction to take toward the food in terms of the angle from the hive with respect to the sun's position in the sky. This angle, of course, keeps changing at the rate of 15 degrees per hour. Amazingly, the dancing bees' angle on the vertical honeycomb in the darkness of the hive keeps changing in accord with the sun's movement if, for example, the dancer keeps on advertising the food source (or a potential nesting site in the case of a swarm moving to a new home) for hours. Similarly, the information-receivers take into account how much the sun *would have moved* if they stayed for a long time before leaving. Their communication involves knowing the time in terms of the position of the sun, both when it is directly visible and when not, when they are within their hives.

Keeping track by an approximately twenty-four-hour internal clock is now known as an almost universal capacity of life, on the basis of what we now call the "circadian clock" (*circa* meaning "approximate" and *dian* meaning "day"). Our construction of accurate mechanical clocks dates back to the days of early long-distance sailing, when accurate time measurements were needed for fixing location (as with the bees) for navigation over oceanic distances. At night, we used the locations of the stars for orientation (as some birds do also). In the northern latitudes we see the stars rotate around Polaris, the North Star (which seemingly stays fixed in place because it is on the axis of the earth's rotation). In the southern latitudes it is not visible, but the north direction can be extrapolated from the location and movements of other stars and constellations moving around it; knowing the time, sailors, and some night-migrating birds, can extrapolate direction.

We are acutely familiar with the truism embodied in the Ecclesiastes saying (there is a time for everything under the sun), yet until very recently we took for granted our ability to predict the time of day by the locations of the sun and the stars and the season by the weather and adjust our activities accordingly. Little did we suspect that a sense of time was needed and routinely applied by other life-forms on Earth as well. We now know that it exists in practically all animals and plants and directs all of life. Each of us has an internal clock that helps regulate our lives, perhaps even influencing how fast we age and how long we live.

Every summer there erupts out of the ground in front of my window a patch of common chicory, a tall plant of the daisy family. Every summer it sports beautiful robin's-egg blue flowers for three months or more, starting in July. Even in its peak flowering time, every morning before bright daylight there is not one flower in sight, but then an hour after sunrise the whole patch is blue with hundreds of opened flowers that by evening are all closed again. One might think that the cycle is due to the light or temperature—that the morning sunlight or warming makes them open and the evening cooling and/or darkness is the stimulus to close them. But a quick and easy experiment proved that that's partly—but not completely—true. I took plants with flowers open at noon and transferred them into darkness in my warm cabin; they remained open till evening and in constant temperature, then still closed at their regular time. Meanwhile, buds (on stalks) that I kept inside in the dark opened in the morning at the usual time, without being subjected to the morning warmth or light. That simple experiment showed that flowers, like the bees pollinating them, have an internal biological clock running on a circadian cycle.

The circadian clock also determines the time of flower death; each of the individual flowers turns from a bright blue to a pale brown by nightfall, then wilts, senesces, and is dead by the next morning, when another flower bud next to it on the same stalk opens instead, to live its daylong life on the plant. Chicory is only one of the many hundreds of plants in the daisy family; others have other very different schedules. For example, the sunflowers in the adjacent garden, as well as common white daisies blooming next to the chicory, stayed open continuously, both day and night, and remained fresh and alive for weeks. Some orchid flowers stay alive and fresh looking for months.

The death and resurrection of other body parts of the same plant occur on much longer schedules. The chicory stalk grows and is alive all summer long—long enough to open all the flowers to be pollinated and produce seeds. Then, by fall, the whole chicory stalk wilts and dies, and over the winter the tall brittle and brown stalks stand and eventually topple, while the roots underground live on to send up new stalks come spring. Thus the plant's life schedule varies from merely a day for the flowers to a summer for the leaves and stalks, numerous years for the roots, and potentially decades for the seeds. Viable lotus seeds have been found in Egyptian tombs, as have viable seeds from the ice ages preserved in Arctic permafrost. Senescence and death sequences are part of the overall adaptive strategy, as are the senescence and death of the leaves of northern trees. The leaves of some trees die and are shed after about three months; the leaves of others remain alive several years.

By February and March, I anxiously await the spring and check the weather report, hoping for a warm day soon when the snow will begin to melt and the brook to roar. In 2020, the leaves and flowers of my snowdrop plants were showing through the snow on April 5. A week later, the poplar trees, the alders, and the beaked hazels had bloomed. Six weeks later, the same snowdrops were still alive and open, while the red maples started blossoming. And so the progression of the plants' blooming would continue with the serviceberry, apple, and blueberry; the basswoods through May and June; the goldenrods in July; and finally the bright blue petals of the New England asters in September and into mid-October.

In most plant species the flowers open within a short period of days, coinciding with the blooming of their neighbors of the same species. In this way, mating occurs (thanks to the pollinators visiting mostly one species at a time) by proxy of the bees and other pollinators acting as male sperm carriers. In their competition for mating agents, such as bees, moths, hummingbirds, and others, plant species' blooming in a staggered, time-specific progression also promotes the plants' reproduction by inducing flower fidelity in their pollinators aside from that stemming from the plants' evolving their flowers to be distinctive not just in their blooming time but also in their come-hither signaling by form, food reward, color, and scent, all acting as sexual reproductive aids.

The trees, the bees, the birds, and humans have evolved to follow not just the earth's *daily* rotational cycle but also its *annual* cycle, which is related to the tilt of the earth on its journey around the sun. One of the first to discover that these long-term cycles are also governed by an internal clock was the German ornithologist Eberhard Gwinner. In the mid-1970s, he used European starlings that he maintained for eight years at a constant temperature and in an unvarying artificial photoperiod of fourteen hours of light and ten hours of darkness. His eight-year-long experiment proved that independent of external cues, the starlings molted their feathers and prepared physiologically for reproduction at nearly the same time each year, despite not having the seasonal cues that those free in the wild did. This annual cycling came to be called a *circannual* rhythm, as opposed to circadian rhythm. The circannual rhythm is, however, thought to be a physiological adjunct to the circadian clock, which by measuring day-length changes (and temperature) determines seasons and synchronizes the circannual response to the seasonal cycle in a manner similar to the way we set the time on our clocks. For animals there is also a season to mate; this is when food availability, determined with respect to the plants' schedules, is greatest and thus when the young offspring will have the food they need to grow. Animals' adaptation to the changing seasons requires long-term preparation by laying up food resources, generating antifreeze, growing insulation, and migrating or hibernating.

This pattern of long-term, approximately yearly, cycles of behavior and physiology was later found in bird migration patterns, in the physiology and behavior of reproduction, and in the hibernation of mammals such as ground squirrels. Under constant temperature and in an artificial photoperiod of twelve hours of light and twelve hours of darkness, ground squirrels still enter hibernation approximately every twelve months. In their natural habitat, this period (repeated unit) is on average but not exactly twelve months, but it is reinforced by or synchronized with the seasonal patterns of day lengths or temperatures, indicating that the circadian clock as well as temperature reset the circannual clock. The duration of daylight measured by the circadian clock is a cue that keeps the circadian clock on schedule with "real" time.

The circannual rhythm is at times tricky to determine, because sometimes cues from the environment, such as temperature, override the circannual rhythm. I notice it almost every fall here in Maine, when both wood frogs and spring peepers start to call briefly when the days get short, as they also do in the spring when they emerge from hibernation. The wood frogs, which close to the first day of a major snowmelt rush to their vernal pools to mate and lay their eggs, already had the eggs ready in the fall and have them kept in cold storage all winter long in their bellies, under the snow. Other cues may be just as or more important. For example, at the proper photoperiod, doves are potentially able to breed, but, as has been shown in the lab, they will then react physiologically (and behaviorally) only if they see a potential mate wooing them and also find material to build a nest with. Similarly, frogs' breeding response quickly stops and the animals proceed into hibernation as soon as the temperature drops in the fall.

We don't know much about humans' circannual cycles. As far as I know, nobody has volunteered to subject him- or herself to a long number of consecutive years of strictly controlled conditions to test for it, nor would we know what variables to measure. Semihibernation and/or running enthusiasm might be a candidate. I find myself loath to run in the winter, although that may be due mainly to the snow and not so much a circannual clock phenomenon; I can more readily go outside when a warm sunny day comes along, but if the next day it's snowy I may stay inside again. I suspect these behaviors could be a remnant of the Neanderthal tool kit, like that of northern bears, of surviving through long Pleistocene winters, where saving energy when food is scarce is a crucial survival skill.

As with the daily cycles of activity, however, animals' annual cycles of migration, growth, hibernation, and reproduction serve well to prepare them for the future. Flexibility is essential, since nature may be inconsistent in the short term. Those that are locked too tightly into a program can face lethal consequences or miss opportunities. Balance and the flexibility to achieve fitness are the products of natural selection. They include animals' hugely varying but distinctly species-specific normal life spans, ranging from a few days to years to decades and up to hundreds of years.

2

Life Span and Aging

THE NATURAL AVERAGE LIFE SPAN OF A BLOWFLY MAY BE A week or two, that of a mouse a year, an Asian elephant's fifty years, an African elephant's seventy, and a human's perhaps less than eighty. In general, the most active organisms have shorter lives, which puts trees at the top of the longevity list. "Methuselah," a bristlecone pine in California, has been aged to 4,850 years, and worldwide several other trees are even older, including an oak of some 13,000 years. However, by far the majority of the trees in my forest live less than a year or two, making the *average age* of the species less than a year, because only one of perhaps hundreds of thousands of seedlings is fortunate enough to grow in the light and thus to survive beyond the tiniest seedling stage. Of those that do reach the light under the normally shaded canopy of their parents, lifetime is hugely extended. However, the maximum age varies greatly, depending on whether they are "canopy" or "understory" specialists. The latter generally grow faster but then live the fewest number of years before senescing and then being overtaken by those that can endure with little light for a long time, taking advantage of time and fickle fate for a chance in the future.

In my forest, the pin cherries live to only around twenty years, the sugar maples more than two hundred. The pin cherries, which colonize clearings, must grow fast and produce seeds quickly before they get overshadowed by black cherry, sugar maple, beech, ash, and oak. For most trees in the temperate region, the clock controls the annual senescence and death of their leaves. Unlike trees, animals are highly active most of their lives, except for a few of the slowest-growing living in cold or nutrient-poor environments. The oldest found so far is "Hafrun," a clam (*Arctica islandica*) that was dredged off the coast of Iceland at the venerable age of 507 years. The annual growth ring in its shell showed it to have been born in 1499. (It was killed in 2006 to count those rings.) Other well-known "cold-blooded," slow-moving animals include turtles, the oldest known being a Galápagos Islands giant turtle named Jonathan, now aged 188 years. Like the clam, he didn't get to be that old by following a regular schedule of running or other exercise. Some of us may try to achieve longer, healthier lives by doing just that. I may be one of them with respect to health and happiness. Good health and absence of disease will of course prolong life. Running has not made me immune to aging, although it has increased my quality of life.

Many of us don't run for fear of wearing out our body from stress, perhaps thinking we have an allotted number of heartbeats per lifetime, much as the seventeen-year cicada counts off exactly seventeen years of near inactivity deep underground and then, after emerging from the ground, flies and sings vigorously for perhaps a couple of weeks. My heart rate may jump from 34 to over 150 beats per minute when I run, and my father cautioned me in my teens about "running too much." But I've hardly ever quit since then. Like others, I've run almost daily at various times to "get into shape," but it was less to add more years to my life than to add more life to my years.

Either way, senescence is inevitable, and life spans are species specific, as is amply demonstrated in both animals and plants.

In temperate-region plants as well as tree frogs, spring peepers, and some insects, the clock triggers their physiology and behavior to prepare for survival in a frozen-solid death state, whereas for other insects it instigates the death of all adult individuals of the population, with survival restricted only to eggs, larvae, or pupae. In most species of wasps and bees, it induces the death of all males by fall; only the females hibernate and then, a half year later, resume their lives as lively as the year before. Although the male and sterile (female) workers of social bees such as bumblebees live only one year, honeybee queens (egg-laying females) live several years, and ant and termite queens decades. The near death of hibernation, from which resurrection is possible, in many diverse animals is under physiological control. It is an adaptive process, timed by biological clocks, and is relevant to humans, too.

Many of us experience the winter blues. They might be induced by photoperiod or some other environmental factor that has left its mark on us through the inheritance of a formerly adaptive trait. There is no known advantage for them now, but I suspect there once may have been, specifically in Neanderthal humans adapted to an ice age climate. The *Homo sapiens* species came out of Africa and spread north after the ice of various ice ages retreated. Recent genetic evidence indicates that there was interbreeding; many of us have some Neanderthal DNA. Most of us feel more energetic and our moods elevated in the spring, as though awakening from a low-energy period. Three percent of the population suffer from seasonal affective disorder (SAD), which begins and ends at the same times every year. So it seems to me that the logical remedy would be to hole up and sleep all day, most days. But the official treatment instead changes the environment rather than the behavior: it recommends increased exposure to light—a longer photoperiod—the signal used by most animals to regulate the circannual rhythm of activity versus hibernation, the period of sluggishness, apathy, and low energy. We don't know what an arctic ground squirrel or a bear feels on entering its hibernation, but those animals' behavior suggests an exaggerated SAD, one necessary for their survival.

Hibernation is a physiological stage that may in some cases approach clinical death, and it is a geographically linked phenomenon related to food availability. Northern bears fatten up in the fall, becoming sluggish and hibernating; southern ones remain active. In northern North America, chipmunks and woodchucks hibernate; gray squirrels and flying squirrels don't. Red squirrels sometimes hole up underground for a few days in bad weather and then depend on cached food. But there are grades of sluggishness. Deer mice huddle together and lower their body temperature when it gets too cold, staying in their nests. Arctic ground squirrels become clinically dead if it gets cold enough. Their heartbeat becomes nearly undetectable, they are incapable of movement, and their body temperature may be at the freezing point of water. Some northern frogs go to the next level: they can freeze solid and are actually clinically dead, except that they can resume life as before if they are thawed. If we had the wood frog's ability to prevent our cells from breaking by flooding our system with something that prevents cell damage, such as glycerol or glucose used by some hibernators, we, too, could freeze ourselves and theoretically live again. Continuing life works for us with the replacement of organs. Many insects do whole-body freezing and thawing routinely; in the high Arctic some spend nearly ten years just reaching the pupal state, freezing solid every winter, thawing in the spring, and having maybe a week or so of active life during which to grow in the summer. Are they dead or alive in between? There is no scientific answer; the question of when life begins and ends is sometimes more philosophical than biological.

A person who has been suddenly knocked out and submerged in ice water, as during an auto accident, can be resurrected. The near-instant cooling of a knocked-out, nonstruggling person by the ice water stops brain metabolism, so nutrients are not used up by it that cannot be replaced due to the heart's being stopped. The brain cells are not fuel depleted, so metabolic processes requiring fuel can resume later. Such people are, like the woodchuck, temporarily in the hibernation phase or like dried midge larvae, which can be stored when dried for decades and become instantly alive insects when rehydrated. There is no absolute state of being alive. There are degrees of it, from that of the dividing yeast cells in our bread dough to the hummingbird that every fall flies from Canada and Maine to and across the Gulf of Mexico to Mexico and South America, then returns to its northern home in the spring, even before the first flowers bloom, to feed on the sap licks yellow-bellied sapsucker woodpeckers make in sugar maple trees.

A large body is generally too complex to revive from artificial death when it is healthy. But parts can be taken from cadavers and made to live again by grafting, as in plants (though plants, of course, can do better by regenerating on their own). Yet in blood, in wounds, and in the ongoing cell replacements in our gut and skin, we do regenerate in our own way. Some animals, including spiders, crabs, lizards, and octopi, can lose a limb as a means of escaping from a predator, which may, for example, grab hold of a leg or tail and end up with only that as the rest of the animal escapes. This adaptive behavior is paired with the ability to regenerate at least a reasonable facsimile of the lost part. Salamanders and newts are especially well endowed with the capability of regenerating parts that are identical to the one lost, including eye retinas and lenses, hearts, spinal cords, and jaws. Since this can be done repeatedly, the animal is, at least theoretically, potentially immortal, provided its parts are replaced.

No mammal can regenerate a limb, but we can heal injuries and regrow muscles, bones, skin, blood cells, and brain tissue. If we lose a limb such as a finger or a hand in an accident and take it to a surgeon in time, it can be grafted back on. What we can't regenerate surgically but only through our own healing ability is internal microdamage. Aging is a slow accumulation of cellular injuries resulting in the deterioration of the body that we call senescence, as a result of which an adult normally dies very gradually at some usually predetermined species-specific time. This process is in the realm of molecular biology, involving DNA and adaptation.

Aging was long thought to depend on the rate of metabolism, a deduction made from the theory that larger animals, which in general live longer, have a lower metabolic rate than small ones do.

Most adult insects that fly and expend huge amounts of energy live only a few days, whereas the larval stage, when energy expenditure is minuscule in comparison, may extend over several years. Mice and small birds have much higher metabolic rates than we and other large mammals and large birds do, and they also grow to maturity much faster. But a high metabolic rate such as that of mice and birds can also be generated in large animals by exercise and stress, and it has been further inferred that both increase the rate of aging. That model was promulgated by Hans Selye in his experiments on his theory of General Adaptation Syndrome (GAS), also known as Selye Syndrome, in which the alarm response was induced in animals at will. It was done in lab animals by accelerating their metabolic rates through forced continuous running or subjecting the animal to cold to increase its metabolic rate to produce heat. It was known, of course, that slowing down bodily functions, as during hibernation, hugely decreases an animal's metabolic rate and may more than double the life span of some small mammals. Fasting them (feeding them less than they would eat on an *ad libitum* diet) also slows their metabolism and increases their life span. Turtles eat little, move slowly, have a low heart rate, and live long. The message was: Take it easy. Don't stress out or pump up your heart rate, or you'll die young like all the small animals with their fast metabolisms and rapid heart rates. You have only so many heartbeats in you; use them sparingly, and live long.

If that were true, it would be bad news for runners like me who routinely run many miles but good news for the armies of couch potatoes. It was what my father believed when he said he was "concerned" about my running. Although he had bragged to me that he had been a superior runner in his youth, he had subsequently and deliberately avoided running, and lived to age eighty-eight.

Selye Syndrome, which connects the physiology of the body to the endocrine system and the rate of living and hence energy expenditure, seems unsubstantiated. But the intake of food *is* correlated with life span, because mice and various other organisms subjected to restrictions of their food intake have longer life spans. The conclusion that forced food restriction expands life span is suspect, however, because the experiments suggesting it were done on lab animals, and restricting food meant doing so in the context of their being confined in a cage, where they *could not exercise* and had nothing to do but eat. Having a caloric excess might, I suspect, simply mean that they grew faster and reached maturity faster and so had an overall shorter life span.

Contrary to our previous interpretations of Selye's General Adaptive Syndrome, much evidence has accumulated over the last half century indicating that mild stressors *decrease* the rate of aging and *increase* longevity. These stresses are wide ranging, including mild irradiation, hypergravity, cold, heat, dietary restriction, and exercise. The kind of stresses that *decrease* longevity are those sustained at high rates over a long time without opportunity to rebound from them.

Senescence is determined and directed by DNA. But how? A way to see how something works is to create an alteration to find out what happens that is different from the norm. One such example of a huge change related to genetic material is progeria, an inherited disease of human premature aging. It affects young children, making them biologically old at ten years of age; they show all the hallmarks of normal aging and then die of senescence in their midteens or early twenties.

DNA is packaged into chromosomes, whose ends have cap-like structures called telomeres that provide a brake to inactivate them. This inactivation is an extremely important process, since cell division must stop at some point or there will be unrestricted growth of the cells, such as in cancer. Preventing certain genes from being expressed is crucial, and the telomeres keep the chromosomes packaged until they are needed for gene expression. During normal aging there is loss of or damage to the telomeres, and telomere shortening, opening the way to pathology, is associated with aging. However, an enzyme called telomerase repairs telomeres and/or makes them longer again and prevents DNA from unraveling. Telomerase regulates the gateway, allowing access to the DNA of the cells and rejuvenating them, which is required in skin regeneration and the healing of wounds. The cells' specific environment in turn influences the telomerase to act in the correct contexts. For example, in a lizard, the removal of its tail is a stimulus for the animal to return to a "juvenal" state and grow a new one. Similarly, if one amputates a salamander's leg, it grows a new one. Specific cues activate the lizards' and salamanders' DNA in responses to cues generated by that species' natural selection pressures. There is, for example, strong selective pressure for some lizards to have a tail but also for allowing it to be lost—since predators try to grab them by the tail and it is better for them to leave the predators holding a piece of tail than their whole body. A similar scenario in trees is the shedding of their leaves in the fall. Like the tails of lizards, the leaves have a biological function, but they are shed when damage or death to the tree by snow loading is possible and replaced by new leaves later.

There are trade-offs in keeping versus losing parts. In trees, it is always the weakest leaves, those that are no longer "working" and capturing carbon from the air, that discolor and are shed first. Environmental cues such as chemical signals may keep a termite queen's ovaries constantly churning out eggs or cut production off in winter when there is no food. Similarly, exercising is important and may, as walking to a salamander or a tail to a lizard, enable us to repair and maintain the status quo and slow senescence. One would then expect that, for us, there is a selective pressure to repair if not renew leg muscle, to strengthen or rebuild it. But if this is true—and it seems to be demonstrated fact—what does it mean molecularly with respect to *aging*? The short answer is, we don't know, but I will illustrate the notion by applying a mechanical analogy to the cell's molecular machinery.

Our body is an inordinately complex structure made of trillions of little pieces. It's a little like a cathedral of bricks, stone, mortar, glass, and glue put together in thousands of precise operations, all relying on "food," that is to say the raw materials that must all be procured, often from great distances, to build and maintain ourselves. The building process (growth) could be hugely accelerated if the materials were all right there at the building site, the location where the molecule needs to attach. If that were so, it would be one hell of a huge pile, clogging up everything at or near the building site. Suppose, at the molecular level, amino acid A had to be fitted at a precise spot on molecule B and there were all sorts of parts from A to Z lying around. There might then be more of a chance of errors being made as the assembly function is disrupted. Mistakes in what amino acid was used would have consequences down the line in a weakened cornice, maybe a wart, maybe a cancer growing wildly and out of control. On the other hand, if food is scarce, the whole production is slowed down. With the assembly slowed down, the procedure becomes more ordered and precise. Oversupply (overeating) may speed up growth and shorten life span by accelerating the time when decline can begin. On the other hand, a gene that facilitates storing resources (putting on fat), which could lead to obesity in adults, may in some environments (for example, in bears when preparing for hibernation) be an adaptation. Exercise may, I suspect, be a stimulus for synthesis for repair, which is another side of growth and/or rejuvenation.

I recall as a young runner having soreness in my muscles, but I seldom did later. Soreness meant injury and was the body's signal to put the muscle to rest for repairs. More serious and more lasting have been injuries that I have sustained beyond the cellular level. They include muscle tears, a spinal disc rupture, a tendon tear, torn cartilage in both knees. All occurred in my twenties, and all have healed. I once again had a knee problem in my sixties, and the specialist who examined the X-rays told me (after hearing about my extensive ultramarathon experience) that I should take up another sport, such as swimming, that would supposedly not "wear out" my knees. I did let up on my running for several months. That was twenty years ago, and I've set a running record since, after I had asked my doctor what would happen if I didn't give up running and he had replied, "I'd have to take your kneecap off and throw it in the garbage can." At my last physical checkup before attempting to run an ultramarathon at eighty, my doctor listened to my heart, then listened again, and said, "Your heart sounds like that of an athletic sixteen-year-old." My knees felt fine. Many of my close friends my age, who have had knee and hip replacements and have never run in their lives, wish they were so lucky. So perhaps we can "rust out" from nonuse, but at the same time there are many people who live long, healthy lives who have never run, while others who run a high mileage die young. Aging is inevitable in any case; only the rate of it is variable. However, I suspect that healing from a minor injury, all the way to the molecular level, may be a process close to rejuvenation, like the regeneration of a lizard's tail after its loss or the replacement of a tree's leaves in spring.

These local molecular disorders that open the way for regeneration come mostly in bursts. For individual trees or persons, the greatest molecular disorder comes very shortly after we're declared dead. But I posit that that is actually the beginning of great regeneration, because we then enter the life of the forest, including its other plants and its other insects, birds, and mammals. It is a literal conversion of our lives into Charles Darwin's version of his famous Tree of Life, which started somewhere around 3.5 billion years ago as a cell that could divide to reproduce itself, but not always exactly, thus enabling selection and hence evolution to happen, and it will proceed, as far as we are concerned, forever.

Do we as *individual* humans wear out prematurely on becoming adults? It may seem so, because many people my age have not only hip or knee pains but also heart or other organ deficiencies, and allergies, plus sleep and memory problems. As far as I know, I'm still in good running shape, despite being a poster child for one who should be worn out several times over. I've run at least four times the circumference of the globe; been subjected, willingly and often deliberately, to other potential stressors such as being stung frequently by bees and wasps, "eaten alive" by blackflies during the Maine spring and then by mosquitoes, horseflies, and ticks; been bitten by tsetse in Africa; and myself eaten mice and various—not always fresh—roadkill. Yet I have not aged or worn out more than those who have not been subjected to and done those things. I can still run.

For an athlete competing on the world stage against the very best, such as in the Olympics, there is, however, a very narrow window of time to compete at that level of the world's best, most likely between the ages of twenty-five and thirty, or younger. An individual's peak necessarily occurs somewhere between those ages, but if a statistician knew exactly when and knew the peak age for 10 million people, they could calculate the peak age of performance for the average person precisely to the year or even to the day. Yet that which would apply statistically would apply to hardly anyone specifically. Each of us is an experiment of one, and everything depends on all else being equal, which it never is. But what the statistic would show would still be the expected and inevitable decline, one that should guide our individual goals and expectations and encourage us to race the biological clock instead of each other.

I'm generally an optimistic kind of guy, but some things are inevitable. Death is not a thing I like looking forward to, but I must look forward to it if I want to get my licks in, as they say.

3

Racing the Clock

IN HIS 1896 POEM "TO AN ATHLETE DYING YOUNG," A. E. Housman viewed the then-common belief of early death from the exertion of running not as tragic but as worthwhile for the glory it achieved for the runner. He advocated doing our running while young, when we can potentially earn the laurels, because "It withers quicker than the rose."

In acknowledgment of that statistical fact, we divide competitive running honors according to gender and age. There are two major categories, the "open" (those in their prime running years) and the "masters" (referring to anyone over forty who still competes). With greater participation by runners of all ages, we have divided age-related categories into decades and sometimes even half decades. We take the inevitable age differences in our running abilities for granted and adjust our expectations.

The age of sixty came so fast that it hit me with a jolt, and it served as a prod to run more seriously with the goal of trying to beat my age-group record time at the 50k distance. But my knees told me to stop running. The pain persisted for months, and I eventually sought help from both the medical mecca at Fletcher Allen Health Care in Vermont and a specialist in Boston. The 17-by-14-inch X-ray films in front of me now are dated

January 28, 2000, and they remind me of sitting in a doctor's office waiting to hear the prognosis. From behind the almost closed door I heard the doctor explain to two interns, "This will be one of the difficult cases—he is a runner and will not like what we have to tell him." I didn't like it, but I kept running anyway, which made what happened later doubly sweet.

The hard running and training that is required to excel and that most people can't do because it is too demanding of effort and time produces damage to the body. That is what aging does, too. But there is a huge difference between those kinds of changes. The body has repair mechanisms for "getting into shape" when that damage is the stimulus *to repair.* After recovery has occurred and the body has achieved a new norm, a rejuvenation process can occur that takes the body to a higher level than previously existed, produced by having used the slight damage as a building stimulus. On the other hand, when the same stress is applied during the time before recovery from the previous damage has occurred, it produces further breakdown, and a continued cycle of breakdown akin to physiological aging occurs. However, my speculation about the connection of both rejuvenation and aging to running is based merely on logic. It comes from my habit as a naturalist watching nature and developing ideas from those observations that I might later pin down with experiments. Those required in this hypothesis may be impossible because they would involve having available and cooperative people over the course of their lifetimes and having continuous access to their physiological states. I have enough confidence in the idea, though, that even after dropping out at the halfway point of a 100-kilometer ultramarathon at age sixty, I then, ten years later, resumed recreational running and started participating in small hometown 10k races. Even if I could not run fast, I could at least finish a 10k. Finishing in any position but first had never been worth bragging rights to me. But then, on September 15, 2019, I ran the Portland, Maine, Trail to Ale 10k and, as a seventy-nine-year-old, finished in 204th place, and it felt grand. There were more than a thousand finishers; I was first in the over-70 age division, and as far as I could determine, my time (59:20) bettered the Maine record time for my age group. When adjusted for age, according to the publicized tables, my time was equivalent to 31:25. As the evolutionary biologist Federico Calboli from the University of Helsinki wrote, "Stuff is eaten by dogs, broken by family and friends, sanded down by the wind, frozen by the mountains, lost by the prairie, burnt off by the sun, and washed away by the rain. So, you are left with the dogs, family, friends, sun, rain, wind, prairies, and mountains. What more do you want?" I could not want to be more, and I felt glad for what I had done with what I had in me.

My running past the age of seventy still felt like that of yesteryear but was, as Bob Seger sang in "Against the Wind" (if I were to trust my clock, as I must), much slower. Running still felt good, but not because of the nostalgia of trying to revive the past, as in Bruce Springsteen's "Glory Days." It was instead no longer the urgent pounding rhythm I had felt when I was trying to get into sync with Cat Stevens's 1971 "Bitterblue" while running the Boston Marathon, with the words "'cause I've been runnin' a long time" ringing in my mind. I just felt as though the headwind had lessened or stopped and I was relieved and felt my energy had not been squandered. The running had fed on itself and grown and reached in different directions. And as Housman advised in his poem that runners perhaps should race "set, before its echoes fade / The fleet foot on the sill of shade," it felt okay to quit while still ahead. But the urgent question of why our running speed declines and then stops altogether remained. How irrevocable is the decline in our race against the clock? How independent from it are we or can we be?

Average lifetime schedules apply among all plants and animals. Mayflies live as aquatic larvae for several years and as reproductive adults for scarcely another day. These cycles are run by internal biological clocks that are set and reset by external cues in the environment. As per legend, the groundhog may stay in hibernation until February 2, when it is presumably aroused by its circannual clock. But if the sun isn't shining when it awakens, it goes back to sleep, a process that in principle has been proven again and again with respect to circadian as well as circannual rhythms. Lifetimes are also predetermined. Each species has a "program" in which time is of the essence. However, here is my point: evolution has provided us with numerous examples where a program is not only internally but also externally influenced, being controlled by cues that have nothing to do with a specific time duration as such but with what *happens to* the organism in time. Examples are legion, but those of fish, mainly salmon and eels, may be the most dramatic. They are the best known, and they are instructive.

In western North America sockeye salmon grow to adulthood in the Pacific Ocean. Then, when reaching sexual maturity (at a time determined by food availability and not time as such) they migrate inland, making a journey of nearly a thousand miles, swimming up rivers to then mate and lay their eggs. Each does this only once in its lifetime, because after that reproductive event both males and females age so rapidly that the flesh almost literally falls from their bones. Something about reproduction, maybe shedding their sperm and spawn, is the cue that ages and then kills them. On the east coast of North America (and the west coast of Europe) eels also die after reproducing, but first they mate and deposit their eggs in the Sargasso Sea in the Atlantic. The chronological age at which the young eels have eventually grown large enough to return to fresh water, where they spend most of their lives, is not well known since the tiny individual eel larvae are difficult to trace in the ocean's vastness.

Few people keep eels to be able to see what happens when they are prevented from migrating to their spawning place, so we have no idea how long they can live. But one famous baby eel, named Putte, was caught in 1863 by a boy in Sweden named Fritz Netzler. It was then about fifteen inches long and had just arrived in Sweden via the North Sea, having at some unknown time been born in the Sargasso Sea, where all our common eels are born. Netzler kept the young eel in a tank all its life, although it soon stopped growing and remained in its juvenile form, whereas if it had been free it would likely have fed and matured in perhaps two to five years and then left to return to the sea. Putte ate little and lived on and on, eventually dying at at least eighty-eight years of age. It was, however, then amazingly still in its juvenile nonsexual form instead of over four feet long, as would have been expected.

Sexually mature eels, those grown to their full length of four feet, make their one-way journey from inland freshwater ponds and lakes to the Atlantic coast and then on to the Sargasso Sea to spawn. Each female lays a half million to 8 million eggs, and the hatchling larvae then float freely in the Gulf Stream until one of the extremely lucky ones happens, after perhaps drifting many years, to reach a freshwater river or stream, which it then swims up, remaining there until it grows to adulthood, which requires eight to fifty-seven years.

The eels' reproductive phase, in the place to which they

migrate, is achieved by a metamorphosis in which the digestive tract degenerates, the eyes and fins enlarge, and the body fattens to provide the energy reserves that will fuel their journey of thousands of miles, which may take years. Meanwhile, these sexually mature adults stay young until after mating and shedding their eggs. Like mayflies, many moths, some salmon, the "suicide tree" from Central America, which dies after blooming only once, and the red kaluta, a rodent of the Australian desert, eels die after reproducing. Is there, then, an advantage to their quickly aging and quickly dying? The answer is both yes and no.

On average in a stable population, only two young of a pair of eels, resulting from the several million eggs deposited per female, get to reproduce. Which of a pair's millions of offspring will win that vanishingly slim chance to reproduce? Does it depend on their specific fitness? Hardly. By far the likeliest variable is chance, which places selective pressure on the parents to produce the largest number of eggs possible. If you do it only once in a lifetime, you put all you've got into it with nothing held back.

There is likely little if anything the tiny larvae hatching out of a 1-millimeter egg in the Sargasso Sea thousands of miles from a freshwater pond a continent away can do to reach a specific destination, except possibly swimming up current if they encounter fresh water. In the meantime, they are destined to drift passively, relying on that chance for possibly years. The parents that produced the most offspring are also the ones that exhausted all of their bodily resources, and thus the chance of their ever reaching their spawning grounds again is nil. As with eels and sockeye salmon, there is a close correlation in nature between a once-in-a-lifetime chance for reproduction and senescence that applies to both plants and mammals.

In the case of plants, the "suicide tree" (*Tachigali versicolor*) of

Central American old-growth forests blooms (reproduces) only once in its lifetime, when it puts out one massive flowering and then dies. Its death creates a gap in the tree canopy, letting in sunlight in which its offspring can grow, whereas otherwise its seedlings would not receive enough solar energy to get a start. In most other trees under similar conditions, such as the American chestnut trees (*Castanea dentata*) in my forest, the young instead get a huge boost for a start from the large nutrient stores that they inherited from their parents in the nut that launches them into the forest.

The most striking example for mammals of the same principle of parental cost of reproduction applies to the red kaluta, a mouselike marsupial of the Great Sandy Desert of western Australia in which for the males, sex is suicide; they drop dead shortly after mating. The red kalutas' problem is that where they live in the desert, the chance of their surviving between one short period of verdure and food after a rain and another is highly improbable. So a male that fails to find and fertilize a female in the rare short period after a rain will make no genetic contribution by living any longer. There is not necessarily any advantage to dying as such. The main reason they do could instead be that there is little selective pressure to *maintain* the metabolic maintenance of repairs to keep from senescing when there is no reproductive future in which to invest in doing so. It's also what a runner may face in perhaps going all out for a lifetime experience of the Olympics when there is little chance for it to ever happen again. The Australian miler Herb Elliott, my running hero as a teenager, was unbeatable between 1954 and 1960, winning forty-four races in a row, but was done running by age twenty-two.

Natural selection has favored "staying young" for as long as it takes to reproduce and keep on reproducing. If instead eels were on a specific time schedule to migrate in order to reproduce, their ability to lay a million eggs would be limited because there would be no guarantee of their having achieved the size, strength, and energy reserves necessary to make their long journey and to bring along the required number of eggs to have a chance of reproducing. Thus some stay young for perhaps a century if they have to, though they could likely reproduce in only a year or two if given sufficient food. It's not that they die deliberately; it's just that there is no selective pressure to stay alive when no descendants will result from doing so.

What does that have to do with running? Potentially a lot, if my hypothesis is correct. The microdamage caused by running is well known; hence there is some validity in the hypothesis of runners "wearing out." It is also understood, however, that exercise serves as the stimulus for repair, for "getting into shape" or being able to improve performance. Perhaps without discrete damage stimuli, the aging or senescence is so slight and gentle that it's insufficient to cause a response and very gradually builds up to cause "aging." On the other hand, if the stimulus or damage is above a certain level and does not let up, there is an accelerated loss of capacity or "aging." An analogy would be that of a house; left unattended, it will, over the course of time, depending on its size, its construction, and the environment, be infiltrated by dust, moisture, mold, and other agents that will slowly but inexorably disintegrate it. We are alert to change, but even large change goes unnoticed if gradual enough and without reference to what was originally there. However, if for some reason the house is needed and therefore is used and kept in shape, it requires a resident (or mechanism) who, when the house is at a certain threshold of disrepair, notices a difference that triggers the repair response. Tiny changes that are noticed then constitute stimuli that trigger the construction that retards aging through repair. The sensitivity of that resident privy to these changes will determine the rate of the house's decay and the time until it collapses.

Human longevity at first glance appears to be an anomaly, because we do not, by any means, cease body maintenance and then die shortly after we stop reproducing. We may do most of our reproducing, or behaviors that accomplish it, in our twenties and thirties, during our best running years, and then go on to live several more reproductive "lifetimes." Ironically, however, the exception of humans relative to many other species may prove the rule: we live very long beyond and independent of our individual reproductive abilities because we still contribute genetically, though indirectly.

The key to our survival is that we are social. We evolved in small family groups in which we helped not only our offspring but also one another, with an underlying basis of genetic related-ness. Females in small family groups, after nursing and caring for their young, likely passed them on to their daughters and granddaughters, who then promoted their own genetic endow-ments indirectly through that service. This is the opposite of the eels' dropping their eggs into the void, hopefully in a place where the hatched young will survive and grow on their own. In our case, the survival of the parents, and even their parents and their parents' parents, is important. Males help in the same way, but perhaps not to the same immediate extent. Their longevity is se-lected for promoting the reproduction of offspring, as in females, but in this case in another direction. A female's direct reproduc-tion finishes at menopause, when her indirect genetic contribu-tion (in our aboriginal heritage) is over. If she had a salmon's or an eel's physiology of repair mechanisms, the time switch would turn it off; she would die. But her repair switch does *not* turn off at that point, because in the distant evolutionary past, those who aided their grandkids continued their genetic line through that behavior more often than those who did not maintain that connection. Males, on the other hand, have the potential to enhance their direct genetic contribution for perhaps decades longer; they can still inseminate. Indeed, males still surviving long after the female menopause have in the evolutionary sense demonstrated survivability and provide proof of quality for future direct genetic investment. The result is that our biological clock continues to maintain the body-repair mechanism for a very long time because it is a good investment for future profit.

Trees provide a parallel. Once grown, they can keep on flowering and shedding seeds (reproducing) year after year; indeed, some (redwoods, bristlecone pines) can reproduce for centuries, even millennia. As long as they can count on future energy and nutrient input, their slow senescence or long survival is an individual investment in future reproduction. Indeed, their chances to reproduce under some situations increase up to a point the older they become. The older a tree becomes, the better are its chances to reproduce. A tree that has reached the light of the forest canopy achieves a much larger reproduction potential relative to one in the understory. However, the adult tree also hogs the energy from its potential offspring, taking the resources they need. If their offspring were all to be beneath its shadow, there would be selective pressure for it to die, as my prior example of the "suicide tree" suggests. The same applies to some animals, especially the social insects.

The queen and king of a termite colony, once established, under the care and safety of the colony, can keep on reproducing for decades, maybe a half century or more. The termite couple stay young "forever," whereas the reproductive adult mayfly (Ephemeroptera), whose larvae live in fresh water, may live only a day. A day is all it takes to mate and lay their eggs, because the insects are synchronized to leave the water at nearly the same time, which facilitates meeting a mate almost immediately, and the water to deposit their eggs is near at hand. No time for mate finding and feeding is necessary; their energy needs to last for only that day. The queen and king of a termite colony may live sixty years. The queen may lay 35,000 eggs per day, the one male doing all the mating, while the workers, who never lay eggs, may live only weeks. This is possible because of the workers' protecting the safety of the king and queen and feeding them nonstop.

Although humans evolved due to the forces of evolution that operate on all organisms, we are fitted to accommodate specific niches. Our chronological age of senescence is not random, it is adaptive, as in all other organisms. What other organisms give proof of is what is behaviorally and physiologically possible, but to see what is operating in ourselves, it is necessary to first fathom our apparent biological agenda, to see how we are similar or different, and to determine the triggers that set off a process.

Compared to our closest relatives, we are unique in our long-delayed reproductive capacity and our longevity. Since human longevity varies, there must be "something" that affects us individually, but without a standard of the rate of aging, it is hard to pinpoint the factors that determine what effects aging has on us. Perhaps one human variable might be a discrete human standard of our biological clock age: menstruation.

The age of menarche—the first menstruation—varies enormously, from about age eight to seventeen years, and we have data on why. On average, menarche in Sweden, Germany, Denmark, Norway, the United States, and the United Kingdom has been noted to have declined linearly from an average of seventeen years in 1830 to twelve in 1970. In other words, *environment* has been having an effect on our aging (though not necessarily on our longevity; the two are not equivalent due to the variables of diseases, predators, and other factors). We do not know why girls are now physiologically becoming adult, or "aging," faster than at any previous time.

We define menarche as the transition from youth to reproductive adult, much as we define the transition from the larval form to the adult in the eel, or the change from a caterpillar to a butterfly.

In all animals the transition from larva to adult is instigated in the brain in response to specific sensory stimuli from the environment that prompt the release of neurohormones (in us, pituitary hormones) into the blood that then affect organs (specifically the ovaries) that then influence the rest of the body. In the case of menarche, the development includes growth in height, fat deposition, an increase in breast tissue, and pelvic enlargement. In short, "something" in the environment changes us, reducing or increasing the duration of our youth and our time to reproduce. But what triggers this process? We do not know what, but one likely candidate is food.

I felt myself underdeveloped since I was a kid and was much embarrassed by it. When I was a freshman in college, some of the male students could already grow a beard, while I only had a bit of peach fuzz. I was called "Benny," the diminutive of Ben, because I was the iconic eighty-pound weakling. I could have compared myself to Putte, the eel that was kept in a tank and stayed young forever but would have grown quickly if it had been fed more and then released to have a chance to swim to the Sargasso Sea. For me, the time to sink or swim came when I arrived at college. There was food on demand three times a day, all I could eat, fried chicken and hamburgers galore, and freedom at last. The world had suddenly opened up, and I began a new voyage.

My nearly six years living in a tiny cabin deep in a forest in northern Germany after World War II were a bit like those of the eel in the tank—tranquil—and I did not eat much because food was very scarce. We picked berries, beechnuts, acorns, and mushrooms and trapped mice. I remember the thrill of finding a raven-scavenged wild boar with some fat left on it. My father once found a deer recently killed by a dog, and one day he came back with a chicken. Some of my most memorable moments concerned food, especially the chicken. I still remember the curve in the road in the woods that my sister and I walked daily to and from the village school. There religion was a subject, but I remember nothing of it except maybe having to be good to go to Heaven. I was thinking of what Paradise would be like, and I decided it was a place where one could eat fried chicken whenever one wanted. I knew little of wanting "things," except perhaps another species of *Laufkäfer* (running beetle, family Carabidae). I found them in the pit traps Papa had dug to catch mice while he was digging out stumps to sell for firewood in some nearby town. The stumps were the legacy of the trees the occupying British troops had cut down for lumber. The British soldiers had also left behind empty cigarette packages, fancy creations with pretty designs of camels and other magic on them, that some of the other boys collected. I collected *Laufkäfer* instead, indirectly because Papa had been good friends with the British. Years later, when mail was again possible, he corresponded with a "bobby" (cop), one of several war prisoners who had worked on our farm in what Papa called *Westpreussen* (West Prussia, a German province) but that I later learned is in Poland. It is perhaps an excusable mistake, as it would seem okay for me to say I'm from Maine, even if the state later became part of Canada.

I was long, some would say, isolated in this magical forest with scarcely a memory of anything before *die Flucht* (the escape). It was as if I was in the womb of Nature; I had no need or desire to go anywhere, because I knew no other things or places. I had no need to own anything, and I was content. I stayed a virgin until I met my bride in Los Angeles at age twenty-six, having postponed growing up and reproducing until later.

Being at home in the forest from age five to ten and not being aware of any other option except for the ruins of the bombed-out nearby city of Hamburg, to which Papa took me once, generated my love of the place, and I was fully occupied there. It was the only place I knew, and it fascinated me at every step and turn. Every kilometer walk, both to and from school, drew my attention and then held me. There was nothing else—no paper, no books, and no music except that of the birds. There were ant mounds that came alive when I poked them with a stick. There were shiny glittering green tiger beetles running ahead on the sand, a colony of digger wasps that carried caterpillars into their burrows, pink heath in flower with bumblebees buzzing on them. Papa's pit traps yielded daily treasures, carabid beetles of various sorts, each more beautifully decorated in brilliant hues than the last, and he took me along when he checked his traps for mice and shrews, which could only ever be seen in the traps. Those creatures hinted at the innumerable, unknown, unseen, unimagined wonders. The birds were the most fascinating of all. A gray flycatcher nested in a box attached to one end of the cabin. Little brown wrens with stout, stubby tails sang from near the edge of the brook where trout lay under the banks, and one wren tucked its nest into the roots of a fallen spruce tree. It was made of a bit of green moss and had a tiny entrance hole. Poking my finger inside, I could feel eggs. It was all so intoxicating that it seemed likely that tiny dwarfs, whom we had not seen but imagined in the forest dancing under the red mushrooms with their white spots, would appear one morning in the small bowers of twigs covered with a roof of fresh green moss that my sister and I had built for them. The real was not far removed from the even more fantastic imagined. The only constant rarity in my environment (unlike that of the rats, which spent their shortened lives each in their square-foot box full of food for experiments on longevity) was food. In contrast, I experienced pure freedom: food and most of my entertainment was reached through the use of my legs.

4

The Running Start

BIOLOGICAL CLOCKS CONTROL PHYSIOLOGY AND BEHAVIOR, and prepare the organism to express responses appropriate to the anticipated environment more closely. Running is not programmed for expression at any specific age—as crawling may be for a larva versus flying for the moth; swimming for a tadpole versus hopping for the frog—but receptivity and responses to key features of the environment may activate it, and social stimulation is a powerful factor that pushes many of us in developmental directions. I probably didn't give running a thought in the Hahnheide forest, but it may have been automatic given the physical reality of just being there. Now, seventy-four years after leaving, I don't remember running but instead the endless details of what crawled, flew, ran, grew, greened, and bloomed, in no small part due to the social stimulation by my father. I probably ran without a thought, especially over the two-kilometer path through the woods to and from school, and that could also have left a mark. As my sister, Marianne, told me later, "You were always running." She probably noticed because she wasn't.

A dear friend recently asked me, "You are a scientist and a runner. Which is more important to you, your running or your nature interest?" As I reflected a few moments, she said, my eyes opened wide and teared. I had reached far back to my conscious beginnings, at Boröwki (meaning "blueberry" in Polish), the name of our generations-old family home in Poland, of which my parents had spoken so often, and the trauma during the war before we reached the safe haven in the woods of northern Germany, having fled our home forever because of the rapidly approaching Soviet troops. For the adults it was traumatic to be suddenly cast adrift from their homes and identity. Mine was still labile; I had none that I knew of, meaning I could go in a variety of directions, take different roads as a response to then seemingly trivial stimuli of many sorts.

We make our identities if we can. And it is satisfying if they are earned rather than given. In retrospect there is mainly one identity that I felt was earned, and that was "runner." "Scientist" comes close, but through unusual circumstances for me the two became closely intertwined, as achieving one became the means of achieving the other.

In the spring of 1951, we landed in rural Maine, where Marianne and I learned English fast as we continued our schooling. That first summer was, as I remember, like a life in Paradise. People from all around visited our family at any time and always without notice, and all of them were friendly and outgoing. We had no telephone, no electricity, no running water, and we didn't miss them, since we had had none in the previous years. I think we were seen as some sort of exotics, and maybe we were. During the summer Papa wore white shorts, whereas other men wore the then-standard blue dungarees, as they needed to while working in the barn with the cattle and haymaking or in the local Wilton Bass shoe factory and the wool-making and woodworking mills. The women above and below a certain age, including Mamusha, sported red-painted lips and black-painted eyelashes. It was summer, and I went barefoot and bare-chested and wore shorts. It all worked fine until, continuing my long-practiced hunting skill with my *Katapult* (slingshot), I shot a red squirrel and had to rummage around for it in a thick growth of green vines that all too soon turned out to have been poison ivy. My closest companions, each about a year in succession younger than I, were Jimmy, Billy, and Vernon "Butchie" Adams, who lived nearby on a big old farmstead with all the critters that belonged there and a lot more besides. Their father, Floyd, limped as a result of wounds he had received on an aircraft carrier in the Pacific when most of the sailors with him had died in an air attack. He never once mentioned the war. The war was over. It was a happy time and a prosperous one for everyone who wanted to work. We four boys tended the livestock, Guernsey cows for milk, Hereford for beef, pigs for bacon, bantams for eggs, and ducks and geese for eating, along with barnyard cats and a big red-haired dog named Jack. After we'd done the sugaring in the spring and the haying in the summer, Floyd took us boys beelining for honey. Beelining further opened a mind already attuned to insects.

Our main objective with the bees was to have fun in the great outdoors of fields and forest and to bring home the honey. And we did get honey, by exploiting the bees' communication system to find their hives in hollow trees in the forest, without any of us at the time having an inkling of what that system was or might be.

No child will become interested in scientific riddles until he or she first exercises the instincts of exploration and chasing. Given freedom from other societal influences, I believe we are born predators and come closest to that state as children. Predators, whether chasing bees or birds or mice (and I was soon predisposed to chase them all) need to know their prey, and that means getting into their mind-sets, which can lead to having empathy for them. I can still feel the intense desire to have near, to hold, and to touch live baby birds as well as beetles and caterpillars—if not live, then dead. All was, at that time, a wide-open window to a fascination with nature, whether insect, bird, or mammal. But a child needs to catch a thing, to have, to eat, to play with, or to keep as an addition to his or her collection and be able to show it off with pride. And so my love of nature and my connection with it were nurtured in the overgrown Maine hayfields, in the fall among the blooming goldenrods and asters. At my age then, the most realistic future I could imagine for myself was to keep in contact with those marvels by becoming a farmer, like Floyd.

By late fall, Papa had bought a run-down farm a mere mile away on the other side of Pease Pond, where he hunted for bats at night, and us boys fished for sunfish in the day and white perch at night. Here, I saw my first turtle, and a raccoon. I often ran back and forth between our farm and the Adamses' place. A neighbor, Phil Potter, told me years later that "you were quite a sight," maybe because I was always barefoot and would have been carrying a white insect catcher net along with my slingshot. A scar on my foot from a cut by a glass shard still attests to my going about barefoot. I had been checking out a bumblebee nest along the roadside, and when I was attacked, I jumped aside and stepped on a piece of broken beer bottle. Our good friend the local Wilton town doctor Herbert Zikel sewed me up at no charge, telling me how hard it was to stitch the thick-hided sole. Those soles were my bodily memory of running, likely going back to the Hahnheide, where they had already seen a lot of travel, until we had received several CARE packages from academic colleagues in the United States with used shoes, after they had solicited us to send them tracings of our foot soles.

Papa and Mamusha got jobs counting, sorting, and packaging round wooden dowels into square boxes at the nearby woodworking mill in Wilton, our town. The work was far removed from anything they had ever done before; being confined in a dusty, noisy, machine-clanging space became unbearable to them. Aside from picking apples at neighboring farms in the fall, there was almost nothing else locally available suitable to the professional mouse, bat, bird, and insect catchers they were. So they contacted former colleagues at American museums and got contracts for "collecting." One job offer involved trapping gophers in the American Southwest and Mexico for a University of Kansas professor. They went and must have done well, because in his long letters in our correspondence over the years, Papa told me much about the gopher trapping. He had found proof that one supposed species of gopher was in fact two species that did not interbreed and having made the discovery wanted to publish it, but the professor forbade him to do so because Papa had been paid from a grant to the professor. Papa then decided to have no more to do with *that* professor. He quit, and ended up being a bit cautious if not disdainful of professors in general. (That would have ramifications much later, after I became one.) But after parting, he hit the jackpot: he got an offer from Yale's Peabody Museum to make expeditions of several years to collect birds in Africa, specifically in remote regions of Angola.

It was an offer he could not refuse, and off he went with his right-hand woman, Mamusha. That was when Marianne and I were sent to a school for homeless kids. I did not like it but could not complain. Life came. It was the way it was. But I had no notion then that we'd end up being there for six years, until graduating from high school. It was only recently that I found the full story of those times in the file of letters back and forth between my father and mother and me. We regularly wrote long and detailed letters to each other, and they kept mine and I theirs and returned them to them. They concerned mostly what they had found in their journeys, first to Mexico and then to Angola, and I in turn wrote what I had found in the Maine woods. They wrote that they wished to take us home, at least for Christmas when they were back, but they were not allowed to by the school administrators, who did not want to make an exception for us when some of the other kids had no home to go to. There was no opportunity for me to leave even once. But, as at home, I acquired a beehive as soon as I could and spent much time sitting by it, watching the bees bringing in their variously colored pollens. I made friends with one of the teachers, Mr. Graft, who tended the school's beehives. After I found a bee tree, he helped me harvest the honey, and I transferred the bees into my hive that I kept in back of the cottage housing a dozen of us boys and a housemother. Running was for a long time not required for anything and was still out of mind but was with me from a seemingly trivial incident several years back that would now become a pivotal prompt.

One day with Floyd, back home at the farm before Marianne and I had to leave, we all took an excursion up Mount Tumbledown (which is next to where I now live in the Maine woods) to pick wild blueberries. Billy, who was still almost a toddler, was falling behind, and I picked him up, put him onto my shoulders with his legs straddling my neck, and tried to jog carrying him up the trail. Floyd smiled and made a comment that included both running and "Olympics" in the same sentence. He also mentioned a relative of his who had been a "great cross-country runner for the University of Maine."

Apparently, running was not just a means of getting from here to there; it was also something done for its own sake. I was approaching an age when I could see something as worthwhile and being identified with it and then being noticed for it as desirable. I was at the beginning of the social stage of growing up. Moving to the United States had required me to adjust to being a stranger in a new place. Strangers are often automatically excluded and have to earn their keep by finding an area in which they can contribute and become of value. Cross-country running, as Floyd mentioned, would become my entry into American society. But it didn't come quickly—or easily.

5

Nature Bonding and Running

IF THERE WERE EVER GOING TO BE A RESETTING OF THE DEVEL-
opmental agenda, if not the biological clock itself, it would have
happened due to another radical change of environment, that of
being sent off to the school at age twelve where my sister stayed
on the girls' campus and I on the boys' full-time with no end in
sight. As a recent immigrant who could barely speak English, I
was forbidden to write in German, and my housemother called
me "the little Hun." I had as yet no personal identity, and my
attachment was still to the woods. On Sunday afternoons, after
attending the obligatory church service, I escaped there from our
cottage and housemother. I ran to escape from the also obligatory white shirt, tie, and suit jacket we had to wear and went
looking for birds' nests in the spring, and caterpillars in summer.
I built a bicycle from discarded spare parts, practiced swimming
strokes in a pool in Martin Stream, a large brook, and in secret
started to build a log cabin behind the cow pastures, the barns,
and the small sawmill at the edge of the woods. By then I had
read the books by Jack London and Ernest Thompson Seton,
as well as by early naturalist explorers about their journeys into
the jungles of far-off Africa and South America, that were in
our small but excellent school library, tended by a librarian who

seemed to suggest exactly the right outdoor nature book every time I went there.

Books opened other worlds. Our seventh-grade teacher, Miss Dunham, devised one contest in spring to see who would spot the first bird of various species, and another to do the same thing with flowers. I probably won both, but being "nature boy" was no glory. After that I kept notes of the seasonal progressions of birds and trees from year to year through high school in my 3.5-by-5-inch notebook, and consulting it now I can see that in 1957 the barred owl was incubating eggs on April 21; on April 28 the red-shouldered hawk started to incubate its eggs and there were as yet no leaves on the trees.

Miss Dunham read good books to us in class: one about Abraham Lincoln in his log cabin, another about the slaves in the South titled *Uncle Tom's Cabin*. But the one that I remember most vividly was about Glenn Cunningham, a boy who was badly burned by gasoline he thought was water that he had poured onto a fire to try to put it out. He was so badly burned that it was thought he would never be able to walk again, but he became not only a good runner but the USA national champion miler. Running was something lofty and transforming. Lo and behold, when finally, in my junior year of high school, there was the option of trying out for the cross-country team, and I recalled Floyd's words.

That summer I sometimes ran on one of the trails that snaked through the acres of surrounding woods to feel the movement, the exertion, and the pleasure of recovery. Being smaller and skinnier compared to most of the other boys my age, I felt disadvantaged but shored up my self-esteem by signing up for cross-country, a popular fall sport.

For cross-country, we lined up behind a mark on the road,

knowing exactly what we had to do. We'd wait for the words: "On your mark," a pause, then "Get set." Then another pause— and "GO!" An official would click a stopwatch and read off a number as you crossed the finish line. No fancy skill was required that you needed special means or privilege to acquire, nor a certain height or weight. Everyone was measured by the clock alone. *Here* each of us stood on equal ground with everyone else. Here we were judged by what we earned, and it could not be argued away. What you earned was yours to keep.

After a week or two of practice, we had our first meet. It was a contest against the neighboring town's school team, Waterville High. Scoring went by the points each runner earned; the higher the finishing place, the lower and the better the score. The first "man" over the finish scored a 1, the second a 2, and so on all the way to the fifth, a perfect team score being 1 plus 2, 3, 4, and 5, or 15 points. In that, the first race of my life, I came in third for the team and fifth for the race out of twenty runners, and scored 5 points. I turned over my notebook that I had used for keeping track of birds and plant progressions in the spring and from the other end now wrote in running entries. The title of the first page is "Cross-Country. Meats [*sic*] 1957," and the first entry reads "1. Good Will. Waterville JV. Came in 3'rd for team, 5th for race out of 20." Entries for the eight more meets of that season would follow. The meet against Waterville's junior varsity was about on par with the rest, and on the ninth, the season's last, I scored second for the team and 16th out of a race of 105 runners.

It wasn't great, but I'd made the cut. I made no mention in my notes of whether our team had won or lost. It didn't really matter to me, only where I had placed overall. I had made the cut in running against the others but was not yet emotionally with them, since I didn't feel I was making a worthy enough contribution. That social development lagged behind my physical maturation, as it probably should, because one can't give until one has something to give. But here was something to work for—something where the more you put in, the more you could potentially get out. It was enough success for me to think that I might have the potential for more, and my second and also last year in high school, and I presumed running was coming up.

Meanwhile, we all had to work. My assigned chores had, over the previous five years, changed from sweeping and washing the floors and dusting the windowsills to washing dishes to being the cottage cook, then to working in the barns milking the cows. To my huge relief, in the winter I also occasionally helped with harvesting firewood and doing barn chores, including helping to butcher the chickens. Then, by a stroke of luck, I was assigned the dream job: mail boy.

Once a day the mail boy carried the mail in a big brown leather bag from the Prescott administration building to the mile-distant Hinckley post office and back again. Thinking of the upcoming cross-country season, I often ran while carrying the mailbag, deliberately not using a bicycle. "Lefty" Gould, the postmaster, took a shine to me, and as hardly anybody was ever there, he would lean out the little window that separates the postal space from the public space to talk to me. He told me about his exploits in the war. To him it made no difference what nationality I'd been or was or whether or not I believed in Jesus Christ. All he really cared about had been his boxing and having been a paratrooper. He knew I was "the little German kid," sometimes also referred to as "the little Jewish kid." I didn't know the difference, but didn't think either was meant to be complimentary. It was particularly the "little" that irked, especially when I was "Benny." I liked the idea of being some kind of "an athlete." It was being *something*.

In a picture I recently saw of myself among my classmates at age seventeen, I saw a skinny, scrawny kid, one I remembered as having no future in sight. There was for me only the "now," and if it wasn't work, it was finding, looking at, and best of all getting a bird's nest or a caterpillar, seeing an owl or a woodcock sky dance, finding a turtle in a marsh, a fish on the line, a bird in the hand. There was nothing in sight until this, my last year of high school.

In the meantime I had flipped my little nature notebook back over again to record the nature happenings of 1958, which for that year started with an entry from May 3: "Black Duck laying," "Goshhawk [sic] incubating." They were followed on May 19 by "Phoebe eggs moderately hatched. Young crows & pigeons have feathers" and thus continuing with entries through July. Then finally, in September, as a senior, I signed up for my second and last cross-country season. I flipped the notebook again to continue with the 1958 cross-country entries.

The first race was once again against Waterville High, but against the *varsity* team. It was a strong team that had scored well in the state meet held at the University of Maine at the end of the last fall season. That time, in my journal, starting from the first race, I listed not only the names of the first five runners in, regardless of their team affiliation, but also the team score. In that race, the first five runners in were "Heinrich, Veilleax, Jeans, Hawkins and Pierce." Only the first was a Good Will Beaver, our school mascot, who "Works when he works, and plays when he plays." I'm not sure which I had done, but probably both at once because it had been an experience of joy, and it was a huge surprise.

Despite my one point for our team, Waterville still trounced us 21 to 40. The team score was far behind for a dual meet, but my victory had reflected well on the team and the school. I had accomplished a totally unexpected upset, and my teammates were glad. That changed my perspective. I would now feel more and more that what I was doing for myself was also for them. Being on a team of runners meant sharing a common interest and having a goal with others. It became a home of the heart and spirit, one that would provide memories that were not just found but earned.

Twelve more races were to come that season, and now there were expectations of me. Lefty told me that I had been in the paper, the *Waterville Sentinel*. He pulled a newspaper out from behind his desk and showed me. Sure enough, there it was: "Ben Heinrich Wins Again." It was something that nobody could assign, give, or take away. It was well earned, and I knew it. Running is hard, and Lefty, as a former athlete and soldier, knew what hard was. His dream of becoming a world champion boxer had been cut short by his having been so badly wounded in the war that he had lain for months in a hospital with doctors advising him to allow them to amputate his leg. They had told him, "If you don't have it done, you will die." He had replied, "Then I'll die." They hadn't operated. He had lived. He had defied authority. That gave me courage.

My running would, I knew, stop after I graduated from high school. I had never heard of anyone running after that, unless he went to college. There was not much chance of that for me. I could hardly afford the thought. But in a strange and roundabout series of quirky and unimaginable circumstances, that changed after a comment by our high school principal, Winfred Kelly. I had not been a favorite of Mr. Kelly, as he had a couple of weeks earlier chased me in his car, stopped me, grabbed me by the scruff of the neck, and kicked me in the butt. I needed punishment because, as he told Lefty at the post office when he picked up his mail, "The little Kraut kid tried to blow up the bridge." It was news to me, but I knew whom and what it concerned: me and an experiment related to chemistry class.

We students were getting bored listening to one another as the teacher had us read aloud from our chemistry textbook in turn. Before my turn I had passed a note to Faye, a girl sitting near me, asking her if she would "go steady" with me. This was only symbolic, as the boys and girls lived on separate campuses. She signed back that yes, she would. So I was exuberant and, in an intermission from our class, looked into a case in our classroom and found bottles and vials with chemicals left over from perhaps a long-ago chemistry class. I talked with Mr. Russell, our teacher, who told me that if you mix sulfur with saltpeter and charcoal (as I recall), you get gunpowder. I found some of the ingredients and wanted to make a firecracker, and he said, "Okay, but don't tell the principal." I said not to worry, I would not try this in school, and mixed various ingredients, poured them into a small wooden vial, and inserted a wax-coated string as a wick to light with a match. Would it just burn, or would it make a bang when lit? I decided to find out at lunch hour, when I set the vial onto the cement abutment over the brook about a hundred yards from the school building. The coast was clear when I lit the wick. It fizzled for several seconds, and just then Principal Kelly came driving by on his way to lunch. The wick had just then burned down to the contents, and a long blue sizzling flame was issuing from the vial at the same moment that I was running down the road because I had seen his car coming. He caught up to me in a jiffy.

Several weeks later, all was not only forgiven but apparently also forgotten, as suggested during one of the routine morning convocations when we students were as usual worshipping God by bowing our heads and repeating the Lord's Prayer, then being patriotic by standing up and putting our right hand onto our chest while looking straight ahead at the flag next to the podium in the front of the room and repeating the Pledge of Allegiance from memory. All that made me feel strange. I didn't understand it any better than I understood chemistry. It was presumably to make us better boys and girls, but I already loved my country, especially the part called Maine. I loved Nature; it was sort of my god. And now I also loved running.

After the obligatory ceremonials, suddenly there he was, Principal Kelly standing up behind the podium in front of everyone making his usual announcements—only this time they included the fact that the cross-country team had again scored a win and: "Ben won his fifth race; he is now an ace!" That did it. Running had won his heart. I was now "an ace," far better than "nature boy" or anything else I had been before.

The public praise felt so good that I looked ahead to try the impossible and did it, winning the next four races, too. The headline of the *Waterville Sentinel* sports page read "Heinrich Sets New Record as Hinckley Wins." I had won my ninth straight cross-country race as we defeated Farmington State Teachers College 19 to 44. Our guys were far ahead. I had "toured the 2.7-mile course in 14:30, shaving fourteen seconds off" my previous record. And then came the reward: Mr. Kelly later patted me on the back and this time said, "Ben, you are college material." I was eighteen years old, and college was the next step.

My English skills were by then adequate but probably not good enough for college. Grades had often been a topic in the frequent exchange of letters with my parents in Mexico, Angola, or wherever else they might have been. Everything I was interested in was *not* being taught or even mentioned, except a course in carpentry by Phil Towle, our shop course teacher, a Quaker who became a soul mate and wonderful friend. From Phil I learned to love building and making things. They were of wood: bookends, picture frames, a chest. I gave them all away as Christmas presents. Shop appealed to me, and in retrospect I understand why. I was full of energies but felt caged; creating something provided an escape. Phil told me I was creative, and he cared enough to invite me and two other boys to another escape, to camp out with him along the Kennebec River. Here was a different habitat at the edge of the river under the tall pines, and at a cabin I was excited to find the nest of a house wren, the first I would ever see.

Having fun and exploring are primary urges at that age, but there come instances when a question is asked: "What will you be when you grow up?" Papa had suggested I become a physician, on the premise that I could "see the world" by serving as a doctor on a ship. My dream tended instead to be to live on the farm, the one my parents had, where I envisioned myself growing food, hunting deer in the fall, fishing in the nearby ponds and brooks in spring and summer, keeping bees, maple sugaring, and cultivating a hobby such as maintaining an insect collection. I could then be out in the woods at any time, as I had been in my sophomore year, when I had gotten kicked out. That caper was assuredly a wrong decision, but emotion proved strong enough to overpower reason. Luckily, that emotion would later be harnessed into something positive instead: running. After the incident, I was able to stay home for a year, and at the high school in my hometown of Wilton, I tried out for the ski team. I did well in cross-country skiing, which set me on the trajectory to cross-country running.

At times of developmental transition, most animals broaden their horizons by dispersing, exploring, and distancing themselves from their parents, but they still stay within the same type of habitat to which their species has been adapted. We are more fluid. In us, mind is an important component of choice and of behavior. My father was grooming me to someday take on his wasp collection, but I pushed back against it. I had wanderlust. In medieval Europe, it was expected that a young journeyman would leave home for a year or more and explore the world. Going to college would also be a stepping out, encountering new cues, new influences, and new paths to horizons not previously imagined. College might be the ticket. I could learn about Nature and then live back on the farm, surrounded by it all.

I had by then been out in the woods a lot, during all the different seasons and under all the different conditions possible, and I hatched a secret thought of someday writing a book about a tree. I had a specific one in mind, a huge ancient hemlock tree that halfway up its massive trunk had holes chiseled out by pileated woodpeckers into a hollow part where bees flew in and out in a steady stream in the fall, to and from the goldenrods in our overgrown fields. It was a magical treasure, also hosting a colony of carpenter ants where the woodpecker had been excavating in the winter. Caterpillars and aphids fed on the leaves, beetle larvae bored in the deadwood, hairy woodpeckers got the beetle grubs, and crossbills came for the seeds in the crown in the winter. If I lived on the farm, I could maybe spend a couple of weeks every month in the tree and eventually see everything and then write a book on the story of the tree. It would be my life's work and legacy. Yes, I'd write the story of the tree, a whole community within one tree. But of course I would forever stay at home on the farm, just like Papa and families had done for generations back at Borowke in Germany, even after it became Poland. I loved our new farm as though it were a Paradise, and I could not conceive of ever being anywhere else. But that did not mean not getting an education, and so I spent my several just-earned dollars and applied to Yale, Bowdoin, Bates, and the University of Maine in Orono, certainly not for job preparation but to learn.

The rejection letters soon came back—from Yale, Bowdoin, and then Bates. My college would end up being the University of Maine in Orono. It had (and still has) a famous school of forestry. Forests and trees. Wonderful; that would be fine. And further good news: UMO had a great cross-country team. The acceptance letter from UMO didn't mention financial support or running. I almost literally didn't have a dime to spare, and my parents didn't, either. Papa kept a ledger in which he wrote down what he spent for every postage stamp (then 3 cents). He wanted me to do the same so that I wouldn't buy what was "not needed." I could work, and I hoped to get a job. I first applied for a summer job at the nearby Mt. Blue State Park emptying trash cans, where I went to see the manager. "How old are you?" he wanted to know. "Seventeen." "You don't look it," he replied and dismissed me.

6

College Horizons

TIMEKEEPING BY EITHER CLOCKS OR CALENDARS KEEPS US regular and on the beaten path, though not necessarily the green and less traveled one of "The Road Not Taken" by the Pulitzer Prize–winning poet Robert Frost. Whichever way we take, there is always a need to enforce some regularity, as the environment we live in is one of many bumps and turns. Most other animals live as natural-born specialists, and for them as individuals it is a matter of do or die, but as a species they make up for specific deficiencies by increasing their reproduction. We can escape many confines of the clock by taking alternate paths and sometimes by just waiting it out. Although my first try at getting a job failed, another then materialized, largely because I had hunted (and still do) for wild caterpillars. I was especially enamored of the caterpillars of the giant silk and sphinx moths, which were a challenge to find in the field. It is also fun to raise them, as some would pets, and see them transform into what looks like an entirely new life-form. It is cheap and easy to do, too, simply by making a cage to hold them from a piece of old screening and providing the leaves they were feeding on when found.

The connection between fun and profit came from Papa,

because he was friends with the State of Maine senior entomologist, Dr. Auburn E. Brower, whose hobby was moths. Brower sometimes visited us at the farm, and in the evening on an overcast night we would tack a white sheet onto the side of our house and place a bright lamp in front of it. Moths of all kinds would come flying in and land on the sheet. (They are not normally attracted to an artificial light as such, but using the lamp rather than the moon or stars to orient themselves by in flight, they turned and came spiraling in.) I especially loved to see the arrival of the hugely impressive big fat sphinx moths and started a collection of just that group. The sphinx moths are the most charismatic moths of all because their large size and hovering ability made them appear superficially like hummingbirds. Dr. Brower, perhaps seeing in me an eager moth enthusiast, helped me get a paying job as a moth trapper, and so that first summer out of high school I worked for the US Department of Agriculture.

The job required me to drive a government pickup truck all over the far northern part of Maine. Luckily for me, I had recently learned to drive, thanks to working at the Potter farm, where I had driven Phil's beat-up old pickup around the field, collecting hay. Now, in Maine's northernmost county, Aroostook, I set moth traps about a mile apart on one of the few roads. They were for capturing one moth species only, the gypsy moth (*Lymantria dispar*), and they could only be males. Each of the traps had a funnel entrance and contained a pad soaked with the female's sex scent. The males follow the scent trail to the trap through the air and, while trying to find the expected female inside, would get stuck there in sticky glue smeared onto the trap's paper lining.

The point of the moth trapping was to find out where that notorious tree defoliator might have expanded its distribution, so that if moths were found, the Maine Forest Service could then spray the county with DDT from airplanes. At the time, large portions of the northern forest were already being sprayed to control another moth, the spruce budworm. The caterpillars of that species fed on and defoliated spruce and fir trees, rather than hardwoods as the gypsy moth caterpillars did. With sufficient spraying the moths' population explosions stopped. What was not well known yet was that if the moths were *not* sprayed, the populations would also crash, and perhaps sometimes just as quickly and more permanently, because, especially at high caterpillar density, viral diseases spread like wildfire. At lower densities, the populations of parasites such as ichneumon wasps and bird predators were also active. But with spraying, those natural control agents were killed off along with the intended targets.

Up in the north woods, I rented a room in the town of Houlton and had almost no human contact all summer. Working for my government paycheck meant driving all day, a mile at a time, stopping at each trap and getting out, checking the trap, then getting back into the truck and driving another mile—all day long, trap after trap. I wanted to run, to train to make the UMO cross-country team that fall, my freshman year, one of my biggest reasons for being there. So there seemed to be a conflict because my job commitment was for all day. However, I solved the problem by combining running with work; when I stopped the truck at every mile to check a trap, I parked it about a hundred yards before or past the trap, then ran to the trap and then back again after checking it.

By summer's end I had not found a single moth in a trap. But it had been a great summer. I had shown that there was no need to spray for the gypsy moth in northern Maine, could now pay most of my college expenses, and had gotten into great shape for cross-country. (As a postscript, I want to digress briefly on the retrospective lesson on the importance of science. DDT was a vigorously advertised "harmless" universal panacea for bug control but in the long run turned out to be highly toxic, especially in birds' reproduction. If its use had continued, it would have eradicated many species, especially raptors such as eagles and peregrine falcons. I have seen gypsy moth caterpillars every year for the last thirty years in my forest in Maine, but I have to look for them; they are not common, and without any spraying here there has never been a population outbreak of any defoliator, or the many hundreds of other potentially defoliating moth species.)

After a long summer alone, I was briefly home again and anticipating the exciting event: arriving on the UMO campus. Finally the day arrived when my friend and neighbor, fishing and hunting partner Phil Potter, for whom I had done chores on the farm and who had taught me to drive a truck, drove me to Orono and dropped me off at my assigned dorm, Hannibal Hamlin Hall.

First things first: I walked over to the adjacent gigantic field house complex and introduced myself to the cross-country and track coach, Edmund Styrna, a tall man with a broad smile and a short crew cut and a former New England champion hammer thrower. I told him I wanted to run cross-country. "Coach," as we runners and other track*men* (there were no women's track or cross-country teams then) would call him through our four years there, was cordial and escorted me to the "stock room," where I was issued standard baggy gray cotton warm-up pants, a sleeveless shirt, a jockstrap, and a pair of the then-standard black canvas, thin-soled running shoes. In minutes I had suited up and went out for a run on "the course," which started at the

880-yard track next to the field house. Afterward, to cool down, I went up a floor in the field house to the weight room. Football brutes were there, lifting barbells. I had lifted only bags of feed grain for cows and, having never handled a barbell, wanted to give it a try, maybe like one big hefty guy I was watching do it: he bent over and lifted one up with his back horizontal to the floor. I didn't know it could be done that way, so tried it, too. *A big mistake.*

A sharp pain in my back extended into one leg, and I was forced to visit the campus infirmary. Dr. Graves, the physician there, eventually diagnosed that I had a ruptured lumbar disk, and an extrusion of it was pressing on the nerve into the leg. My long-anticipated running career seemed over before it had even started.

There was no improvement for a month despite my sleeping on a board to keep my back straight. It was agony during the then-mandatory (for all male students) army ROTC drills. After a couple of months of no improvement, I was referred to a spinal specialist in Bangor. He had no cure, either, saying that an operation would be "risky." Furthermore, he recommended that I change my declared forestry major to a career in something "not requiring physical exertion." It sounded like a death sentence to my running. But being partially immobilized had a positive influence: it gave me no option but to spend most of my time hitting the books. UMO, the state school, had a generous admission policy, but it was coupled with a high ejection rate that sadly included even my friend who had also been admitted. He had been the salutatorian of my high school class of twelve students.

By Christmas vacation, the pain had started to subside slightly, and when I was home for the semester break, Phil got me interested in weasel trapping. He had done it as a young man in Wytopitlock, in northern Maine, near where he had stayed and worked at a lumber camp cutting cedar trees and shaping them by ax into railroad ties. As a sideline while there, he had trapped weasels, to sell the ermine pelts that were then in demand. He now showed me how to make, set, and bait traps, and how to prepare the pelts. Trapping seemed like a romantic, fun thing to do to get out into the woods that made me feel alive. It required only mild exercise to tend the trapline through the woods and over fields. I risked it, and to my great surprise and happiness my leg pain lessened.

Back on campus for the spring semester, I had a meeting with my faculty adviser, Professor Malcolm Coulter, in the Wildlife Division of the School of Forestry. Professor Coulter was an expert on and researcher of the fisher, a member of the weasel family. I told him I'd been trapping weasels of both common local species, *Mustela frenata* and *Mustela erminia,* and at the same time catching a number of other small mammal species, which Mamusha prepared as museum specimens. Dr. Coulter was interested when I told him about what I had seen and learned from the experience of tracking and trapping weasels; seeing *Sorex* and *Blarina* shrews, *Peromyscus* deer mice, and *Clethrionomys* red voles, as well as red and flying squirrels; and reading patterns in the snow related to habitat. To my surprise he encouraged me to write it up as a paper for a small publication of original science research, the *Maine Field Naturalist.* I did, and to my even greater surprise it was accepted and published while I was still a sophomore. I had titled it "Weasels in Farmington" in reference to the nearest sizable town.

I now had something *in print*! Something with a whiff of science to it. Although running was now again edging forward and had been a big part of the genesis of the paper, another seed with a possible future had also been planted. Now the running was connected with its true mate, biology, the study of living nature. Although I was proud of my paper then, I later removed it from my curriculum vitae in embarrassment because of what I was soon led to believe, namely that biological science was supposed to be molecular, what "Weasels in Farmington" could never be. (However, years later I proudly put my first publication back at the top of the list, finally realizing that direct contact with nature in the field could be, as it had by then become to me, a matter of choice and often the source of the rarest, most original, and sweetest fruit.)

Pressure had built up throughout my difficult and painful freshman year from the frustration of being unable to run. But nothing seems more precious and motivates more than that which seems within grasp and is then yanked away. The running passion didn't go away, even as I studied hard and later worked at various jobs I found on campus. One was in a cafeteria and another in the Bear's Den in the student union building, where we hung out in groups around tables drinking coffee (from real cups that needed to be washed). Most of my efforts were directed at my studies, though, and I earned some B's and an occasional A, both then highly vaunted honor grades. That was not unusual; our track and cross-country teams had the highest average GPA of any group on campus, but I wasn't running. Still, I kept dreaming of being able to run, and by summer I felt the gift, the ability to run, slowly returning. I then applied for and got a job through the School of Forest Resources to again work in the north woods of Maine, but even farther north, in the Allagash region. This time it was with the companionship of a crew of four fellow UMO forestry students, working for the International Paper Company.

Our job was to walk long parallel transects through the forest with a spray can of red paint, to select and then mark trees to be cut by the mostly French-Canadian loggers in our lumber camp. We would squirt one spot of paint at breast height onto the trunk of the tree selected to be cut, so it would be seen by the logger, and another spot at the base to ensure honesty after the tree had been removed by the logger, equipped with his chain saw and horse. We moved forward in a row separated from one another and far enough apart to cover the area to be logged. It was all day, every day, almost constant low-grade exercise. We were free on the weekends, but our logging camp was too far in the north woods for us to be able to visit our homes in the south. I had brought along my small mammal traps and kept myself occupied and earned additional money with a trapline, this time catching mice and shrews to fulfill an order from Turtox, a biological supply company. I caught mainly short-tailed shrews, *Blarina brevicauda*, to be pickled in alcohol for use in anatomy dissection in introductory biology labs. But I was interested in other species, too, and made stuffed museum specimens of them.

After returning to the University of Maine in Orono that fall, I showed my catch to a zoology professor, Albert Barden, a mammologist, who was excited by one shrew I caught. My father was not and accused me of brownnosing. Perhaps he was jealous, as he had not finished a university degree and had not gotten the recognition he felt he deserved from professors. But truth be told, I did indeed get helpful guidance and encouragement from professors and also learned something, and because of that would later switch my major to zoology.

Catching shrews was not my only extracurricular activity at logging camp. Our camp was at the end of an endless dirt road from Ashland that led into the endless north woods. Every day I ran about four miles of it out and back after supper. With no idea of pace, I simply ran according to a degree of effort that felt like work without straining too much. Our daily hiking was not peppy, and it let up even more when our boss, Mack McLain, came to join us once a week from the paper mill back near home in Rumford. When he came, we often all sat down together in the mossy woods somewhere, listening to his jokes and telling our own.

That fall, on the first day back on campus, I again went to the field house and suited up to run on the cross-country course. On that first run I met another runner, the previous year's Class M (medium-sized schools) Maine high school champ, and tagged along with him. On returning, as we neared the field house, he said, "Let's race!" "Okay." We took off. I don't recall much, but he later told me that even while still wearing my boots, because we had not yet been issued our running gear, I had left him "in the dust." That exaggeration had some truth to it: my running had improved over the summer. I had, two years earlier, once beaten Bert Hawkins, the eventual Maine state Class L (large schools) high school cross-country champ from Waterville, but it had not been a true *running* victory. It had been a fluke because he had stopped to take a leak. But this was real: I had kept up with a great runner and could perhaps now, in my second fall, finally make the UMO varsity cross-country team and have a dream come true.

Several days later, after having gotten settled and attended my first classes, I trotted out onto the quarter-mile track again to meet Coach, who was there evaluating potential runners for the upcoming cross-country season. He had been a New England champion "weight man" at the University of New Hampshire in his specialty, the hammer throw, and now had to deal only with cross-country runners, a different species. He greeted me with a big smile. It was good to be back, and it felt great to be able to run. "How about a mile, Ben?" he asked.

"Okay, Coach." I lined up. "Ready, set—go!" he called and clicked his ever-present stopwatch. Running on the *track*— wow!—I felt smooth and light in my new black canvas running shoes. I loved the feel. I'd have to run only four laps. Easy. Finished, and Coach clicked his watch again. He looked at it. "Four-thirty!" he said with a grin on his face. I wasn't particularly tired. "Want to try it again?" Sure. And so, after several minutes, I did it again, and then one more time, one after another in almost the same time. Coach beamed.

Sad to say, although everyone else's speed improved through the season, mine did not; maybe it even declined. We never did speed work in cross-country (running short distances at a fast pace—for example, repeating 400- or 800-meter intervals with short rests in between). The total mileage I ran with the team went down. I did as other members of the team did, which was mostly to stay together. I did not try to push ahead of the others. I just made sure not to fall behind. Cross-country races are distance running, but only of about five to six miles at once. That means slowing down a lot relative to running a mile or half mile. Slow running was what we seemed to be practicing, and there was no argument or discussion about what we were doing and how, because we became the best team in the state, with dreams of winning the Yankee Conference title the next year.

The athletic banquet where we were served a big steak dinner in a crowded hall was also the occasion for choosing the next year's team captains. I remember only one moment of that event, Coach standing onstage by the podium, unfolding pieces of paper, one from each member of our team, with our choice of captain for next fall written on it. I was potentially a candidate because I had kept up with Mike Kimball, the acknowledged best distance runner in the state. On three occasions I had caught up with the first-place finishing teammates of the race and had deliberately not passed them. Why should I? I was on a team, and it made no difference in the scoring which of us came in first or second; we would still score the same 3 points. During that year, I had made a miraculous recovery from my back injury and had developed a deference to each and every teammate with whom I felt strongly connected. We had battled hard. We had won and lost but mostly won. We had come together as one. During our trips to off-campus meets, my teammates had asked about my accent and my past, an interest that made me feel connected to them. I ran, as one said, "like an animal." I had found my home in running. *I was of and for the team, the only group I'd ever felt close to.* One after another, Coach unfolded the little papers and tallied the count, one that contained my slip, but not with my name on it. I could not practice self-promotion in a vote that concerned the team.

Coach rose slowly, straightened up, paused, looked over the audience with a serious expression, and announced, "The captain for next year—is Ben." I was overcome with emotion. Finally, I had been accepted for who I was by those I felt closest to in our common cause. But it would all too soon turn out differently than I had hoped.

My parents were going on yet another yearlong expedition to Africa. It would be, as both they and I knew, their last one ever. Papa told me so. He was getting old, and he looked and felt it. Mamusha had almost died on their last expedition to Angola, and she was not even sure she would join this one. Now they needed me, and it was my one and only chance to be with them, as well as a once-in-a-lifetime adventure. I'd be damned if I went and damnable if I didn't. So I went, despite feeling guilty about letting my teammates down and especially knowing that they would be unable to understand.

I was away in Tanganyika (now Tanzania) for a year spanning two summers, when I otherwise would have been working and earning a paycheck to cover my college expenses. During this experience, my hardest and most demanding job ever, for Yale University, I didn't earn a dime. For me, what was even more costly was that I had to stop running. I was to be a hunter of mostly small, secretive jungle birds and a taxidermist of them in the afternoons and into the evenings, every day without exception, along with Waziri and Baccali, our two native African helpers of near my age, and my mother. Our catch, a communal product, is now encased in the scientific collections of the Peabody Museum at Yale.

My personal African running experience was brief. I had run laps on the deck of a freighter, *The African Moon*, on a monthlong trip from New York that included a diversion to a port up the Congo River, plus other ports along the east coast of Africa, and then on to Dar-es-Salaam, our destination. Once there, while we waited for weeks for our truck to come in from the United States (so we could take it into the wilds of isolated mountain island jungles), I ran on a dirt road at the edge of the city and met up with a fellow runner, who took me to a local all-comers track meet. I ran the two-mile, and a local cowherd lapped me on the 800-meter track. Much later, in the interior, I outran a large spitting cobra as it chased me after I had stunned it with bird shot. I was in occasional contact throughout the year by letter with Coach in Maine, who told me that a Kenyan studying at Cornell had won the IC4A Championships running bare-foot. So at the first opportunity in what is now Arusha National Park, I tried a barefoot run myself. All went well until darkness started catching up to me. I was still far from my pup tent, my mobile home that year, and, fearing lions, elephants, rhinos, and Cape buffaloes, had no option but to keep on running. It cost me the soles of my feet, and I could not walk on them for two weeks. However, the elephant dung beetles that I caught as a bycatch would bring me back to Africa several times many years later, after my PhD in biology, opening up new chapters not only in insect physiology but also new ideas about and insights into the human biology of distance running. Nevertheless, getting back to Maine after fifteen months and reuniting with my UMO cross-country and track mates was one of the happiest days of my life.

I had been a skier in Maine as a senior in high school, winning every event at a tri-school winter carnival, and had broken the medial meniscus of my right knee after skiing just for play several years later, when I owned a car and after some downhill runs at Sugarloaf Mountain resort needed to push it to get it started. But much earlier, Coach had convinced me not to go out for the UMO ski team, to avoid possible injury for running, and instead run indoor track in the winter (and then spring track). I took his advice and earned three varsity letters per year and regularly ran the two-mile race, winning the state championship one year. It was in the spring and the event was at Bates College, a half-hour drive from home. Neither my father nor mother ever showed up at any of the track or cross-country meets, but I never expected them to and so of course could not miss them. But Phil Potter showed up and sat in the bleachers for the state championship meet on a glorious sunny day.

Years earlier, Phil had taken me on many hunting, canoeing, and fishing trips all over Maine, and I had worked on his and his wife, Myrtle's, farm earning the money to buy my first camera and my first gun, a single-shot Remington .22. He would eventually give me his own .30–30 Winchester lever-action rifle, with which I shot my first and last deer. It was during the year I was home because I had gotten expelled from the Good Will School for running away. Phil now came alone and sat in the first row in the bleachers at the Bates meet, right next to the tracks that we two-milers would circle eight times. For most of the race I was trailing Mike Kimball, my senior in more ways than one. Mike, the best distance runner in the state, who would later set the US record in the longest distance run in one hour, had two or three laps to go, running a few steps ahead of me. Phil jumped up from his seat and started cheering like a banshee. He had never been to a track meet, and as I was battling toward the finish and slipped by Kimball and then won, Phil jumped up, so excited that he barfed up his lunch. My time was not impressive and is neither remembered nor worth mentioning, but neither was my UMO field house two-mile record attempt. To leave a trace at that institution, which I admired so much and which had become a home, would have been an honor. It was an all-comers meet where I decided to give setting a record in the two-mile a serious try. It was my last and only chance to do so, and I had trained on my own, according to how I felt the work should be done.

The meet was in the winter, in the familiar field house, where you have to run many laps on the indoor track to add up to two miles. For many such lap races, officials designate the starting and ending points and make sure the runners complete the required number of laps, signaling the beginning of the last lap to the front runner. With one lap to go, the leader or leaders can then unleash with all that they have left. I was on pace for the record and knew it, just waiting to hear the *bang* that would make me fly. When it sounded I took off, running like never before, knowing that was *it*, my last race at UMO ever. But then there was another bang and then a third!

The two extra shots, as I soon learned, had been meant for me to *stop*; the race was long over. The official had messed up and had not given me the last-lap signal that I had expected and had waited for. I had already finished, having missed the record by perhaps two seconds due to saving my kick for the lap *after* the race had ended. I could have beaten the record but didn't. A fellow teammate, I heard, passed it a few years later. There are running rules; that's what makes the sport inspiring and the running great.

7

On the Science Track

MY FATHER HAD PERHAPS BEEN RIGHTLY WORRIED ABOUT MY running too much. There was no visible future in it for me, and I was graduating. Now what? At least one thing was certain: I now had freedom and could exploit it. It was time to take stock, and while browsing the university newspaper I happened to stumble on an ad about a very cheap student charter flight to London and back that summer. On impulse, I used the cash I had earned washing glassware in a lab at the university, bought an air ticket, and ended up spending two months cycling all over Europe, of which I had heard about so much but seen virtually nothing except our tiny forest retreat in the Hahnheide.

An hour or two after landing at Heathrow Airport, I purchased a used bicycle, crossed the English Channel on a ferry, and started pedaling off to Paris to see the *Mona Lisa* in the Louvre. I carried no baggage except an occasional bottle of red wine and a loaf of fresh bread, and I slept in youth hostels for a couple of dollars a night. After Paris I pedaled north to Oslo to see the Holmenkollen ski jump, where Olympic events had recently been held, and also visited the Viking Ship Museum. Then it was back down to Hamburg and from there on to revisit the tiny cabin hidden in the Hahnheide where I had spent a large part of my childhood. To my surprise and with a deep emotional rush, I encountered there on the path to the cabin, now barely visible, an object of my earliest love, a *Laufkäfer* (running beetle). In total surprise I broke down and sobbed with joy, perhaps at the sheer magic that had happened since I'd traveled over the same spot more than a thousand times and seeing the old cabin standing unaltered, except that the window was now shuttered. The door was unlocked. Alone in the forest, with no human footprints near, memories then awakened. They were of beetles, bees, birds, caterpillars seen and held, and individual trees that I still recognized. I stood long at the willow tree by the since-obliterated path that led over the brook where we had felt under the bank with bare hands to catch trout. I saw the fork in the alder tree where a pair of long-tailed titmice had made their baglike, lichen-covered nest. It seemed like time was reversing, like I was revisiting the past. It was a renewing and strengthening of a deep and already long trajectory of a life in the life sciences, one I had started to leave behind.

Biology had started to mean, I thought, spending a lot of time with test tubes in the lab or identifying new insect species and giving them clever Latin names that would make sense only to those who could speak that language. Latin had been an academic requirement in high school, and I had done poorly at it. Taking biochemistry at UMO and learning how proteins, carbohydrates, fats, and nucleic acids are constructed of carbon, oxygen, nitrogen, and hydrogen atoms and how the structure of the DNA molecule was not just chemicals but a literal script of information that is duplicated in every cell and explains some aspects of inheritance, evolution, energy expenditure, and nutrition had been fascinating. However, most of this seemed out of reach in everyday experience. After returning from the year in Africa I had switched from majoring in forestry to biology, when I discovered that I didn't need to take Latin to become a biologist. However, I hadn't found a path in the labyrinth of possibilities.

One of the first courses after general zoology (biology) that I had signed up for when I had switched to zoology at UMO was physiology. It was taught by Professor Charles Major. He studied rats, and I recall his telling us how he operated on them and removed their livers (or parts thereof), which would then regenerate. Apparently, the rat's body knows it needs a certain-sized liver and then makes it. Professor Major wouldn't try the experiment on us. That was what rats were for, he said, to use as models. You could do with them what you could not do with students. He could, however, test our lungs by having us exhale into an apparatus to measure our lung capacity. When my turn came to blow into a calibrated tube to see how much air I could exhale, he brought the class to attention. "Look," he said, "Ben, a runner, he'll have a huge lung volume in comparison to Josh here, a smoker." He was trying to either educate or moralize. But it backfired: my lung volume measured less than the smoker's.

In science, as in running, all comparisons are in terms of the presumption of all else being equal. In biology, everything is time-bound; what happens now depends on what happened before. Reality changes almost moment by moment. So all else is hardly ever equal. Biology is complex. It's not like nuclear physics or astronomy, in which a mathematical equation to describe a phenomenon with precision is universal, independent of time. Perhaps my lungs were smaller. Perhaps I had inhaled with less effort, or maybe my lungs were so efficient that they didn't need to be as big to do the same job. Maybe lung size increases to compensate for inefficiency. I was starting to wonder about age, too.

Most of the runners I knew stopped running before they were twenty-five or thirty, as though in accordance with an inviolable biological clock that dictated that one had a limited number of heartbeats allotted for a lifetime, and since running caused the heart to speed up three or four times the usual rate, one could use those heartbeats up either slowly and live long or fast and die young. My father had run in his youth. He was a health freak who had never smoked, drunk a glass of beer or wine, eaten peanut butter, or run another step after his brief youthful flurry as an event-winning runner. He had advised me not to run for those reasons, but I was not convinced that my biological clock would speed up and make me age faster and die younger. I didn't know and wondered if I was still able to improve. There was only one way to find out, and that was by studying the biology of aging in relation to exercise, perhaps in biochemistry, and then seeing near the end, in perhaps an experiment of one.

In one class, professor Ken Allen gave us the assignment of proposing a problem of physiology and then designing experiments to solve it, then doing as the faculty did, writing a research proposal to secure funding from the National Science Foundation. For my topic I chose exercise and titled the work "The Biochemistry of Diet and Exercise in Relation to Aging." It came to six pages of handwritten blue-ink text that I still have, fifty-five years after having written it. Reading it now feels as if it had been written recently, because despite the volumes of research that have by now been carried out, there is still so much we don't know.

I began my report citing the way a scientist, Clive McCay, had already in 1930 showed that restricting the food intake of lab rats in strictly controlled scientific conditions greatly retards the appearance of physiological functions and aging. His data were solid. It appeared as if, with all variables held constant except for food, food was an aging agent, if aging is defined in length of life span. One might thus be tempted to starve oneself to try to live longer. Another scientist, Hans Selye, had later, in 1950, proposed that exercise *decreases* longevity because it increases the "rate of living," implying that we "wear out." In my report I suggested that in all of the animal experiments concerning food's effects on aging, the variable of exercise had not been controlled. The rats had been captive in small cages for the researchers' convenience. Nor had the effect of the duration of growth to achieve adulthood been factored out. Exercise burns up calories. At what time does aging begin? Or perhaps humans do not react like lab rats; it seemed to me that the results of experimental animals in small cages were irrelevant to the question. Perhaps rodents in little cages are bored out of their wits and simply eat way too much because they have nothing else to do. They did not need to run to reach food as they would normally in nature, so perhaps they were dying young from lack of exercise, and perhaps also from growing too fast, or from boredom. Maybe exercise is like a nutrient such as salt, a lack of which is life threatening but a lot of which can kill. Part of the answer to the decreased longevity of the lab rats may, I suspect, be provided by an unplanned experiment on humans, conducted many years later.

Starting in the early 1980s, we have had what looks to be an epidemic of drug abuse, alcoholism, suicide, chronic pain, obesity, and reported unhappiness. The underlying cause could be frustration with the ever-changing, ever-more complex demands created from increasing dependence on expensive and complex devices that are becoming needs, not options, of modern life, aside from ever-higher taxes, helplessness in the face of robots replacing people, and fewer jobs that promote or involve self-worth for ever-larger portions of our population. This dire trajectory has been explored in the book *Deaths of Despair and the Future of Capitalism* by Anne Case and Nobel Laureate in Economics Angus Deaton. I suspect that the symptoms are similar to those of the caged rats in the experiments because both the rodents and the people have no way out, and with ever less to do except feed off the always-easy-to-reach food that would normally require active search in the wild in contact with Nature, much is removed from life that is normally provided as a matter of course. Having no need to do or possibility of doing what they are designed for, both mice and men will miss physically and psychologically what they are made for and, having thus been placed into an unnatural situation, experience a lack and suffer the loss of a normally routinely psychological and/or physical nutrient. We do have the ability to live better and longer. However, in contrast to the lab rat in its cage, we can find escape with the use of our legs and our minds.

As a runner and dyed-in-the-wool biologist, I was of course interested in medicine. Medicine concerns curing a body that has something wrong with it; like fixing a car, that can't be done until you know how it works and what makes it run. So I applied to medical schools after having taken the Graduate Record Examinations and scoring in the 99th percentile. I suspect it might have been because I had written in the required essays on the applications that I strongly disapproved of the then-current practice of X-raying the bellies of pregnant women. It seemed unnatural and thus harmful. I got a uniform response: rejection.

With still no resolution, it seemed prudent to at least get my military obligation out of the way. To buy time, I went to enlist in the army. Enlisted men could choose their assignment. I had chosen the paratroopers, to be stationed in Germany. But there I was rejected also, on physical grounds: my record showed a serious back injury, the ruptured lumbar disc. What was left?

That was when I turned to graduate school, first in a continuation for another two years at UMO in the lab of Professor James R. Cook, who earlier, while I had worked there as an undergrad washing glassware, had allowed me to take a leave to go to Europe. He now offered to take me on as a master's degree student, where I could continue much of what I had been doing anyway; plus he let me join him in his research on cellular metabolism, and I still got paid. Our collaboration felt as though I'd been lifted to the clouds. It felt like a real-life rerun of Sinclair Lewis's novel *Arrowsmith*, which I was then reading, in which Martin Arrowsmith becomes an assistant to a professor he greatly admires.

Professor Cook was my Max Gottlieb to a T, and he led me, during my two years as his student, to three scientific papers in leading journals, on the metabolic pathways *Euglena* cells use to process either glucose or acetic acid (an ingredient of vinegar) or how they survive without any carbon source other than carbon dioxide from the air, with energy from light for photosynthesis. After my public defense of my completed master's thesis, presented in our auditorium, the professor came up to me after I had finished, pulled the ever-present pipe from his mouth, and declared, "That was the best damn seminar I've heard here for a long time." I was awarded my degree with distinction, a huge and unexpected honor but one I felt I hardly deserved because just about everything I had done I owed to his guidance. Ours was a work of love, for its own sake. We had in our collaboration both understood the same thing. He now advised that I broaden my horizons, go someplace new, and get a PhD. Charles Major, our physiology professor, suggested the University of New York at Buffalo, where the authority in the topic of respiratory physiology, a professor named Hermann Rahn, taught.

I applied and was invited for an interview so the people there could look me over. Entering Rahn's office, I noticed a mouse swimming underwater in a covered fish tank. It never once came up for air, so a lot of air pressure must have been applied to the water to increase its oxygen tension so the mouse could extract enough of it to exercise. I was impressed and waited patiently and politely for the professor to begin the conversation, since he had invited me. But he just sat silent and looked at me. Then, after a few minutes, he got up from his chair and abruptly declared, "This interview is over." I guessed it was and went to see the next professor I was scheduled to meet. That gentleman was chatty and asked me why I wanted to become a biologist. I told him the story of how, in the Hahnheide one sunny spring day on my way to school while crossing the brook where we had captured trout by hand, I had looked up into the big willow tree because it was abuzz with big furry black and rust-brown bumblebees visiting the flowers and—"You," he declared before I had finished, "are a naturalist"—implying, I thought from his enunciation of "naaaturalist," that he meant I was not really a physiologist, and was therefore unlikely to ever be a scientist. I hadn't even mentioned my undergrad publication in the *Maine Field Naturalist*, "Weasels in Farmington." In retrospect, in my naivete I had downplayed what was then of huge academic significance. Biology was in the midst of a tremendous revolution; it was the beginning of the molecular age, due to the stunning recent breakthrough by James Watson and Francis Crick of the University of Cambridge, who in 1953 solved the riddle of the molecular structure of the DNA molecule, establishing it to be a right-handed helical structure of two chains of nucleic acid molecules wound around each other. When the DNA unraveled during cell division, "something" was read off the then exposed DNA molecule to produce specific sequences of the twenty available amino acids into proteins, each one a very specific sequence of millions of possibilities that all life is made of. From that, the first and perhaps most critical question boiled down to, *What is the code?* Some research had established that it was likely a sequence of three "letters" or bases on the DNA (and the RNA copy of it) that coded for each amino acid on the protein chain, so that the precise sequence of bases carries the information to make entire proteins. But what was the code? There was a frantic race in biology at that time to crack it. Excitement was high, and in my interview for PhD study in Buffalo, where I was pegged as a naturalist applying for entry into the halls of the science of biology, I should have known that only three years previously, on the night of May 27, 1961, Heinrich Matthaei helped open the floodgates of the new biology when he saw the results that would make history.

As elaborated in exciting detail by Matthew Cobb in his 2015 book *Life's Greatest Secret: The Race to Crack the Genetic Code*, on that night Matthaei (in the lab of Marshall Nierenberg at the National Institutes of Health in Maryland) saw the results of his clever experiment of nearly a year to crack the DNA code. He had created a protein in a test tube, a chain consisting of *only one* amino acid, phenylalanine, using a nucleic acid chain (mimicking DNA) of *only one* base, uracil. He revealed that RNA (a copy of DNA) uses three base molecules of this specific kind (UUU) to code the amino acid phenylalanine into the chain of usually many different amino acids strung together, as in the letters of a word. In effect, he made a fake mRNA (messenger RNA) that then made a protein consisting of a chain of only one amino acid. UUU was thus revealed as the first "letter" humankind had decoded in the genetic code. The discovery paved the way to the codes of the nineteen other amino acids used by DNA to write the books of Life, knowledge that now allows us to read the genetic script, and it has revealed the common heritage of all of us on the tree of life.

It was a heady time, and I was not knowledgeable about these fabulous wonders and their magic implications. With all of Life on the academic menu—how it is created, what it is, and how it works—there was little enthusiasm for a beetle catcher and bumblebee watcher. My interviewers' near contempt of me, a naturalist, aspiring to become a scientist, was an understandably legitimate sentiment. I had no inkling of the huge potential prizes in the offing, awarded in the often fierce races and competitions for specific research goals that can beckon from a major discovery.

As I slunk back home to Maine and told Professor Cooke about my disaster at Rahn's lab at the University of New York at Buffalo, he looked thoughtful for a bit and then pulled the pipe out of his mouth and asked, "How about you go to UCLA?" "Dick" (as I then called him, after we had collaborated in the *Euglena* respiration work and had gone on fishing and hunting trips together, along with other zoology department professors) then talked about how to advance my work at the DNA level. Ideas were emerging that the chloroplasts of our *Euglena* were in fact derived evolutionarily from a *separate* organism, perhaps a single-celled alga living as a benign parasite inside that protozoan, and by extension the microorganisms evolving into green plants. The mitochondria that drive the energy expenditure we were measuring in them were potentially of such a symbiotic association also, one with ancient bacteria. We had no means in our lab by which to study these exciting possibilities, and I had thought of Los Angeles as perhaps the last place to go. But now suddenly going to California and UCLA was adventurous. "I'd love to!" I told him. And it was done. I was accepted without an interview and with an offer of a salaried research stipend to work on a PhD project of my choice.

Stepping into the unknown can be and often is exciting. It can also be scary. It was both of those for me at UCLA, where I started in a DNA lab, meeting the lab's three other already well-advanced grad students. I was to them undoubtedly an acknowledged rube, one straight out of the Maine woods. For the first time living in a city and alone at a giant university, I knew nothing and nobody. At a meeting I went to for new international students, I met Kitty Panzarella, a sweet and friendly student of Italian descent who lived in nearby Anaheim. We soon fell in love. I think it was right after I got her a beer; she had asked me to buy her one at the counter because she, an undergrad, was underage.

My new sponsoring professor, Thomas James, who had accepted me, was no longer in the lab. He was in the main office, as department chairman. I was from day one academically on my own, and it took me almost half a year before I acknowledged that I was not making discoveries in my professor-endorsed study of protozoan DNA. This was not like running, where I knew what to do and then did it. Even after a year, I was still clueless about what to do with some of the DNA that I did manage to extract from protozoans. I had to drop my prechosen project, that of separating the DNA of *Euglena*. With my PhD chances looking ever dimmer, not even catching a glimpse of anything, never mind nailing down an experiment for a possible scientific discovery (which I had learned is *the* main requirement for a PhD in science), I developed mysterious joint pains. First I had been running well on the UCLA track, then was just walking, then on crutches. A doctor I consulted could not explain the cause. It was not arthritis, and my blood had no signs of uric acid, an indicator of goiter.

I had not wanted to quit but needed to get away from something; I was not sure what to do, except perhaps to set off on an entirely new life-giving trajectory. My solution: after abandoning DNA, I joined another lab in the basement, where faculty and students tended toward whole animals, birds, reptiles, and mammals and their behavior and physiology in relation to adaptation to environment. So now in California, after quitting DNA, I reveled in a coastal marsh alive with nesting avocets and green tiger beetles, and the Mojave Desert with its ravens, jumping mice, and lizards. Among its many other marvels, I even found sphinx moth caterpillars feeding on jimsonweed. I had raised such caterpillars in Maine as a kid, and now at UCLA brought them into the lab and raised them on fresh tobacco leaves from potted plants (tobacco grown by botanists next door for experiments on a virus). I became curious how the huge grub-like caterpillars consumed leaves several times their own body length without moving from one spot, perhaps also using the huge leaves as a sun shield to save themselves from overheating and excessive water loss. But how could they use the leaves as a sunshade while at the same time consuming them? Did they just eat more and faster to make up for the extra water loss? Did they have a mechanism for conserving water after depleting the leaves of one of the widely dispersed plants?

The caterpillars' solution to the first question was elegant and came to me easily, with relatively few simple observations, experiments, and measurements, and I quickly published it as my first legitimately scientific paper, in the prominent British journal *Animal Behaviour*. But trying to figure out how they maintained their water balance in the desert sun and heat was more difficult. I experimented endlessly and found nothing that was not already in the scientific literature. However, the moths that the caterpillars yielded became exciting; they could fly *without overheating* from their heavy exercise of over sixty wing-beats (muscle contractions) per second. How they could fly in the California summer desert heat without cooking themselves in the process was a puzzle worth pursuing.

It was well known that many insects heated themselves up to prepare for physical activity by shivering, but being small they lost heat rapidly and thus cooled in flight. It was logical to presume that they produced just enough heat to achieve the body temperature of choice, as we do. But from the measurements of their metabolic rate in flight that I was then making, it was clear that they had the *same* heat output regardless of what air temperature they flew in, and since their muscle temperature also stayed relatively steady over a wide range of air temperatures, they had to have a mechanism of heat loss, one that stabilized and regulated their body temperature. But *how* they did this was puzzling, because they didn't sweat, as we do.

I eventually narrowed down various possibilities and began to suspect that they used their blood to shunt heat from their hot flight "motor" to the abdomen, which then acted like a car "radiator." My then new professor, George Bartholomew, was in Australia for the year studying mammals, so I was (still) on my own. But his replacement, insect physiologist Franz Engelmann, whose specialty was the juvenile hormone as studied in cockroaches, gave me a rude nudge. When I told him my hunch, he simply didn't believe it. He told me that to prove it I would have to remove it, meaning the circulatory system. Ha! Fat chance. But the closer I got to my moths, the more I saw, literally—especially after I removed some of their covering scales and looked through their almost transparent, clear plastic–looking cuticle, the exterior skeleton—the possibility of proof, one way or the other, by a definitive test using a strand of my head hair.

I threaded the hair with a surgical needle around the tube-like "heart" wherein blood is shunted from the abdomen (where there are no muscles producing heat) to the moth's front end, where the muscles powering the wings are located. I took these operated moths into a temperature-controlled room, set them down, and waited for them to shiver and warm up, then to fly. Those flying in a cool room flew well and continuously, whereas those in a warm room crashed to the floor in a minute or so, with vastly overheated flight muscles. Those results paved the way to proving that the moths, upon reaching a flight-muscle temperature only slightly higher than our own, start to transfer the excess heat created by the flight exercise into their abdomen, which then acts as a heat radiator. It was beauty of the finest kind, and it was for me a lot more exciting than if I had won the Boston Marathon. I immediately wrote up the experiment, along with the tests of the alternative hypotheses, to publish in the research journals, including two for *Science* and two for the *Journal of Experimental Biology.*

The results applied to exercise not only in the heat. In an experiment regarding the opposite of shutting off the heat-dumping mechanism, I tested for the moths' ability to *reduce the heat generation* necessity for flight, where, in an analogy with a runner whose steps suddenly become magically light, I gave the moths that option of easy or low-effort flying with greatly reduced energy expenditure (and the heat production associated with it) using a simple apparatus in which they were suspended and could fly continuously in circles while a sliding electrical contact allowed a running (flying) measurement of muscle temperature. The moths thus suspended on the flight mill were suddenly very light in weight and then coasted along expending just enough energy to continue flying. It was no great surprise but nevertheless revealed that they kept flying at the same altitude (they had to because they were suspended) but now produced much less heat. No longer was there excess heat to get rid of, and they stopped maintaining a high and constant flight muscle temperature.

My sudden and unexpected scientific breakthrough had come soon after a period of intense frustration, during which I had started the physical deterioration that ended my running on the UCLA track. The mysterious joint pains at first seemed like evidence that perhaps we *do* wear out, because the pain became worse, until I had to walk on crutches. But at age thirty that quick decline was not the likely cause of the trauma. My apparent wearing out had not been due to too much running and reaching the end of some biological clock allocation for running, even though most people stopped at about that age. I believe it came not from physical stress but rather from the mental stress of feeling lost in more than one way, in the (to me) void of the city, the new alien culture, and the utter frustration of my work. But after the *Eureka!* experience in the research breakthroughs, the pain soon stopped as if I had simply turned it off.

Meanwhile, Kitty Panzarella and I had married, and we had taken almost annual cross-country trips back to my parents' farm in Maine during the summers when I was studying bumblebees. The medical problem had then vanished, even when I was chasing individual bumblebees (identified with differently colored and numbered tags) on their often repetitive foraging routes. I then resumed casual running on the road. Nobody else ran then, as far as I could tell. People looked askance at me running down the road in shorts. I was "a sight" then, and they'd toot their horns when driving by. Once an old UMO classmate slowed his car down next to me, leaned out the window, and asked incredulously, "Are you *still* running?" No, it was more like *again*. I felt reborn, as though I were restarting the clock.

While deeply engaged in my PhD research, I had had no contact with my new major professor, George A. "Bart" Bartholomew. He had generously accepted me as a graduate student within a month or so of leaving for his sabbatical year to live and study mammals in Australia. But Bart had gotten me onto the right track by suggesting I make a list of six potential PhD projects before he left, which had me at first stuck in the library and then out into the nearby Anza-Borrego and Mojave deserts looking for something to study. The caterpillars and sphinx moths were among a few less promising possibilities out of which the moth project had blossomed as if out of nowhere. I suspect it came in no small part because I had long been enamored of these moths and had collected both the caterpillars for fun since a child and the moths in my hobby collection.

I was now, after all the exciting results, anxious to tell my professor about my new research, and finally did so at a temporary research station in Papua New Guinea, where he was studying bats. It was near the end of his one-year leave from UCLA in Australia when he had invited me to join him in New Guinea because, as I had informed him, I was an experienced jungle bird and bat catcher, skills honed during my undergraduate-year leave to Africa from the University of Maine.

In New Guinea, I helped catch both bats and birds for his studies, while continuing to take body temperature measurements of both tropical butterflies and sphinx moths. I don't remember seeing or hearing any great excitement about the New Guinea bats versus those from Australia or California, but when I told Bart about my results with the sphinx moths his eyes widened. He stood still. I was struck by his silence. He seemed in thought, and then after a long pause he offered to fund me for a year on a postdoctoral fellow salary off his National Science Foundation research grant. Then I went silent. I was in a quandary. What to say?

I didn't yet have a PhD, and still had to process some of my data on preflight warm-up, which was valuable because it strongly supported my previous exciting discovery that contradicted prevailing dogma. He had no problem with this: "What you have done with caterpillars is already sufficient for the PhD degree." I disagreed. It was insufficient. But who was I to argue with my professor? My moth exercise physiology research was by far more valuable than anything I had done with caterpillars, and I wanted my PhD to be on the moths' flight exercise physiology, *not* on caterpillars' leaf-feeding behavior. Still, I accepted the postdoc offer, and he suggested that we write my data on moths' energy expenditure while shivering to warm up to fly together. That made sense, because body temperature regulation of birds and bats was his trademark research topic.

Being hugely pleased to see his interest in my moths, I also told him about my bumblebee studies during my summers in Maine and about the obvious implication for other insects: that surely the giant dung beetles that had so impressed me in Africa were as, if not more, hot blooded when they came zooming in to partake of elephant dung piles, and furthermore that large moths would have lower body temperatures despite their size, *provided* they had large wings so they could partially glide along in flight and save energy, unlike the high-speed sphinx, which are like fighter jets in comparison. It worked: he sponsored *us* traveling to Costa Rica, and then to Kenya's Tsavo elephant park, to do those studies. He even supported my projects on the botanical implications of bumblebee foraging on pollination ecology, asking if I minded if he talked about the energetics aspects I had told him about at a scientific meeting. Did I? Of course not!

In the meantime, after arriving back at UCLA from my summer work with bumblebees in Maine, my postdoc was suddenly shortened. Franz Engelmann, my PhD cochairman, told me a job opening for an insect physiologist had come up at nearby University of California at Berkeley. He was the one who had told me to do the impossible to prove my theory: eliminate the blood circulation, and I had done it, by a hair. I had told him no, I did not want to apply for a faculty position in Berkeley. His response: "You'd be a fool not to."

I applied, and was accepted to immediately begin an insect physiology teaching/research faculty position. But there had been a funding crisis, and the Entomology Department had not been able to provide the equipment needed for the job it had promised. That turned out to be a huge opportunity, because I had a backlog of data on the behavior of bumblebees in a pristine bog of native plants in Maine. It all needed to be mentally digested and transferred to script, and I was sure the work had worth, not only in terms of studying the physiology of energy use but also because it concerned the bumblebees' role as ecological agents in plant community structure and plant evolution. The link hinted at an explanation of the fabulous variety of flower forms, colors, and scents, and the differences in their reward kinds and schedules of nectar and pollen. It explained why flowers had *not* all evolved according to one "best" or optimum model but had instead acquired huge *differences* in those features even while luring the *same* flower-constant pollinators. Similar ideas were becoming rife at that time, but there was not much data. They were discoveries of a theoretical kind, but they were discoveries nevertheless, and worthy of data for support or refuting. I spent a lot of time writing a paper for *Science* on the topic, but after about the seventh draft trying to get it just right, I decided it would be a good idea to get an outside perspective, preferably from someone in that area of biology.

Bart suggested I talk to another professor at a nearby university, who he thought would be interested. I was eager to please and to receive feedback on the paper I had written and rewritten again and again on the topic. But I still wanted to run it by peer-review before sending it out to the journal *Science*, for which I had formatted it. And so when the professor invited me to come talk to his class of graduate students about it, I felt honored and did so promptly.

The event turned out to be electrifying; I sensed excitement. The topic was apparently right on, and as I was leaving the building, the professor came out, walked up to me just as I got to my car, and asked if *we* could publish a joint paper on the topic. *What?*

I was stunned silent for a moment, then declined. He offered to help me secure a grant. I still declined and told him I had already rewritten many drafts of a paper. Could I show it to him? he asked. Of course I could, and I gladly mailed it to him, anticipating the usual comments, criticisms, corrections, and suggestions. But the response shocked: my previously typed manuscript had been rewritten in his own handwriting and then sent to bigwig National Academy of Sciences members in that field of expertise, who replied to *him* that they liked *his* exciting idea. (More than liked, I later presumed, because both he and my major professor were elected to the National Academy of Sciences, the highest honor bestowed in the United States for original science research.) All that was fine and wonderful, but I felt cheated—I could no longer publish it by myself. How could he *not* be coauthor; the paper had *already* been distributed to scientific peers, who when seeing it again as peer reviewers, if I were to submit it now, would then assume I had stolen his ideas. At this time he was organizing a scientific meeting on the topic. I learned of it and wrote one of the other organizers to ask for an invitation, and so attended and presented, showing data relevant to my thesis, which he then in a public address there described as "incoherent," adding that I had "extended the ideas of Bartholomew" when it had, in my opinion, been precisely the other way around. However, nobody does anything without what they consider a good rationalization. I had one when shooting at wilted ferns thinking they were a deer; our brains are wired to invent "reasons" to justify what we want to do. He had asked someone I know: "Who does he think he is?" I was a mere unknown assistant professor, perhaps someone to help and facilitate by his name.

I felt totally done and done in. It was painful, and I seriously considered quitting science entirely right then and there, despite my very attractive faculty position at UC Berkeley, where I got on well with every one of many wonderful, friendly, and helpful colleagues. My work was acknowledged and I "advanced" almost prematurely to full professorship. But eventually I decided no, I would not allow myself to be manipulated nor leave on the basis of hurt pride. But leave I knew I would. I belonged back home in Maine.

I stayed at UC Berkeley for ten years, all the while continuing the annual summer migration to Maine with my wife, Kitty, daughter, Erica, and dog, Foonman (and once also with two young ravens). Overall it had been one the best experiences of my life. Due to my light teaching load I could explore a new trajectory that led to exciting comparative physiology, behavior, ecology, and evolution. It went from the hummingbird-like sphinx moths' exercise physiology to that of the physiology of bumblebees, which was the same. At times the bees conserved most of the heat they produced in the thorax, as during foraging, while at other times they dumped the heat into the abdomen as the sphinx moths did, except that they applied the same mechanism to incubating their eggs and larvae (by way of their abdomen), despite an anatomy that looked designed to prevent such heat loss. How could they, I wondered, be anatomically designed to save energy to conserve the heat needed for flight muscle operation in the cold, while also being able to transfer massive amounts of heat to their abdomen to incubate eggs and larvae in the nest? Solving the riddle meant having to look inside the bees and observe the behavior of their various internal parts. When I finally solved the puzzle, the data presentation required twenty-four figures published in the *Journal of Experimental Biology*. That paper was for me the finish line, the breaking of the tape, at the end of a very long struggle after which I felt I could breathe again.

The work had involved simultaneously measuring the bees' breaths and their pulses of blood circulation. Pulses of heated blood were shunted in opposite directions at either the same time or alternately. When not in a countercurrent mode, heat from the outgoing blood was recaptured by the ingoing blood, and when they were alternating, heat transferred out of the thorax and into the nest. The bees' breathing was synchronized with their blood-flow pattern, using the air spaces in their abdomen as a bellows, like a cheetah's bounding, in which the chest cavity acts as a bellows to facilitate expiation and inspiration in synchrony with the bounds.

From the animal studies I became conscious of something similar in my running. When my strides were smooth and unlabored, they were synchronized with my breathing; two steps (one each leg) were coupled with one inhalation, and the next two steps with one exhalation. Increasing stride length and/or an incline changed the ratio: at rest there are two heartbeats per one inspiration there, and the same for the exhalation. The breathing/heart/step ratios change or are abolished when working hard, as my heart rate rocketed from my normal 35 to 40 beats per minute to about four times that rate desynchronized. I took that to heart, when considering the trade-off of efficiency for endurance versus power for speed, to choose a relaxed pace for endurance when they would be maintained so that one interferes the least with the other, to help enhance overall efficiency by reducing energy cost.

Running ability may be as complex as the bumblebees' flight and as natural if trained. It is one of, if not *the* defining difference between us and our closest living relatives. It is written in stone by our forebears' footsteps, now fossilized in volcanic ash at Laetoli, in the Great Rift Valley of Africa, where australopithecines left running tracks that are almost indistinguishable from those of *Homo sapiens* almost 5 million years later. We are born runners, which makes us unique among the now-existing hominids. (Nor can we now claim superiority over the apes as "the toolmaker," nor from all other animals as "the thinker.") Our footsteps are a record not only of behavior but indirectly also of body form. I compared my own running versus walking tracks made in light snow. The match with those of the preserved pre-human tracks imprinted into a thin layer of volcanic tuff looked perfect. Those ancient hominids could indeed have run (as well as walked), and there is no reason to presume they did so much if at all differently than we runners do now.

Pondering our own sensitivity to cold, our lack of body fur, our shock of thick head hair, and especially our ability to sweat profusely, it is abundantly clear that we both are born to run and originate from a hot climate. If we could have, with one swoop, eliminated our sweating response, as I eliminated the sphinx moths' ability to get rid of their exercise-generated heat with a hair, we would have been eliminated from the cradle of our evolution, the open plains of tropical Africa.

Our prodigious sweating response is a strong indication of an ancient heritage of not only living in a hot environment but also having a home base in it, for the simple reason that we would have needed to drink water in order to sweat. And to drink water, we had to be near a reliable source of it. Examples of the need for access to water are evident when we look at insect thermoregulation. I know of only two insects that regulate their body temperature using evaporative cooling: the honeybee, *Apis mellifera*, and the desert cicada, *Diceroprocta apache*.

The first collects nectar from flowers, which is typically nearly 90 percent water, most of which must be evaporated in order to become honey. So with their nearly constant "problem" of having too much water, the bees use it to cool themselves in flight. The desert cicada plugs its mouthparts into the phloem of trees and bushes in the desert and thus taps into water deep in the ground via their roots. It therefore has no problem achieving heat balance in places where other organisms that are unable to reach that water cannot live.

I had invested many more hours, effort, and emotional capital into my science than into my running. It is, like science, a lonely sport, and it is for individualists. The 100-meter, the mile, the 10k, the 100k, and the 100-mile hold magic. They test performance and quality, cleanly, simply, and truly. There is no doubt that the 100 meters tests speed. There is no doubt that a 100-mile race tests stamina, the ability to go the distance. The requirements—and the results—are clear. There is no ambiguity.

The clock says exactly where you stand, and only *you* can decide where and how far you can or want to go, and it gives back to you what you put in. John L. Parker, Jr., would say it best in his novel *Once a Runner*, in which the character Denton says to his friend Quenton, "Let me tell you something about winners and losers and other mythical fauna in these parts. That quarter-mile oval may be one of the few places in the world where the bastards can't screw you over, Quenton. That's because there's no place to hide out there. No way to fake it or charm your way through, no deals to be made."

8

California Running

AFTER RETURNING TO UC BERKELEY IN THE FALL AFTER A SUM-
mer in Maine, I met Max Mische, a tall, rugged, long-haired running dude of natural exuberance, on the tartan track at Edwards
Stadium on campus. We were marginal hippies, both imports
from the East and dyed-in-the-wool runners. He was escaping
from his roots and family in New York City, while I was doing
the same but from the Maine woods. It was the 1970s, when love
was supposedly free and Jim Morrison was blasting the airwaves
with "Come on baby, light my fire / Try to set the night on fire . . ."
We were aglow. And not just with running. I, too, was part of the
Flower Power movement—but in the Berkeley lab with summer
bee projects in the fields of Maine: a *literal* immersion in flowers.

Forty-three years later, Max and I reconnected and caught
up on our Berkeley running. I then learned for the first time that
we had traveled parallel paths, not just then but since childhood.
He, too, had been a *Flüchtling*, one of the millions of escapees
from one enemy or another in Europe during World War II. His
family had been driven out in an ethnic cleansing from their native village of Altlag (in Gottschee, a region of German settle-
ment for seven hundred years) in what is now Slovenia (then
part of Yugoslavia, after Hitler and Mussolini had invaded it

in 1941, putting all German minorities there at great risk with the communist Partisans who were fighting the German Army). The village was destroyed, and the mostly German people of the village had been forced to leave, losing everything. His family had ended up in Austria, where Max had been born in a refugee camp. In 1952, the family had come to Brooklyn, his soon-to-be-beloved home, where he had grown up attending a Catholic grammar school. In high school he had excelled at running and been elected captain of the track team. At almost the same time as I had, he, too, had been struck by wanderlust and headed west to California, where we had met.

Max wrote me in 2020:

> I can vividly recall, as if yesterday, how one afternoon you came loping down to the Cal track with a copy of *Scientific American* in one hand and your track spikes in the other. With your bumblebee article with a big bee featured on the cover, and this, I believe, marked the start of your profound quest into nature's mechanisms and strategies related to the animal world. I am certain that your passion for running and ceaseless investigations into the natural world fed into one another, adding fire to each.

Informal academic groups centered on specific disciplines would meet in seminar rooms on campus, but an informal group of us runners that prominently included Max had also formed on the UC track. We met at noon or late in the afternoon to run. Mark Gruby, an older gentleman and former sprinter and horse trainer, became our self-appointed mentor and coach. He critiqued our running form: arm swing, leg lift, even the positions of our thumbs were subject to correction under his critical gaze in an effort to perfect the art and science of the race against the most important variable as measured by his ever-present, ever-correct, never-judgmental stopwatch. Speed through smoothness was the goal we all aspired to. Max had both. In body type he tended toward that of Alberto Juantorena (known as "El Caballo," the horse), the Cuban running phenomenon who had won both the 400 meters and 800 meters in the 1976 Montreal Olympics and who was then as powerful in our imaginations as Usain Bolt would become some three decades later.

I was hoping to catch up with Max and others of our loyal and always enthusiastic running group by doing regular repetitive speed work, late in life for developing peak performance as it was for Max and me. But it went better than expected. In my 1974 running logs I read with joy and satisfaction of our daily ritual of running intervals of 220s (yards), 330s, quarter miles, half miles, each of usually three to five repetitions with quarter-mile to two-mile jogs in between. We challenged and encouraged one another, and we routinely ran our 440s in under a minute. I reduced my former best quarter-mile time at UCLA by three full seconds, to 54.0. Three seconds for that distance is a lot, and that achievement brought up a new thought: Might I be able to run a two-minute half mile? My best time for that distance, three seconds shy, was not even close, and the barrier now loomed as a target. Then, on October 29, 1974, I ran a timed half in 2:00.6, missing the magic mark of the two-minute half mile but coming close enough to taste it, after having run the first quarter in 57 seconds. I could see my mistake; it had been my pacing. My running notes read, "Tied up last 220. Next time do first 440 in 60.0. *No faster!*"

The guys knew I had been thinking of someday breaking the two-minute barrier in the half mile and decided my dream had a chance. They wanted to give me a little help and arranged to stage a private event where Mark would officiate and Rick Brown, our UC Berkeley star half-miler, would pace me as rabbit. I was more excited about racing the clock than I had been for any race. I remember lining up one Saturday morning when the track was clear, the stadium empty, and Mark releasing us from the starting line. I ran the first quarter following Rick, holding back slightly, as planned, finishing it in exactly a minute, as planned, then letting rip and finishing in 1:59.4, a mark I still keep as a remembrance.

Mission accomplished; it was the last half mile that I ran in a race, and the best. I was a distance runner among sprinters and middle-distance runners, so the speed success was a big deal to me, and in no small measure it was a team effort with my running buddies, Max, Mark, Rick, Glenn, and the rest of our Berkeley track mates.

After that I spent less time at the track and entered races such as the UC intramural Turkey Trot at Thanksgiving, where the prize for winning would be not a trophy or a time but a turkey for our family: Kitty and Erica, our young daughter. Sometimes I would jump into all-comers meets where I entered everything in sight, up to four different events per meet, including the javelin throw, before eventually eyeing the marathon as a logical finish to my running career. It was a year or so before I left the state of California and its Anza-Borrego and Mojave deserts and redwood forests that I loved, finally submitting to the lure east of the sirens of the Maine north woods. But the friends and the excitement of California would forever be a cherished experience.

Max, "the Poet of the Track," had sent me another email in October 2018, a beautifully enunciated statement of what it is to be a runner that recalls these years:

As the years rush by I, like you, Bernd, hold ever dear those resplendent running days we shared once on the Cal track together, and in whose shadow we struggle on, knowing what once held us close will never return. We raged wild and free once . . . on those brilliant sunny days on the Cal track, where for just a few seasons in our youth in the 1970s, heaven knew our names. Feeling that sudden rush of aliveness and ecstasy, we sensed it could not last. Yet, back then, our small band of runners, joined together in that ineffable magic, had seemingly escaped the bonds of time and mortality. We were powerful runners once; and it haunts us still. We are among the blessed, having known a beatitude that remains in our hearts and souls. Grateful we are for "the sweet time, the golden time" (as you once called it).

Few will ever know the rapture that came to us through running. We were the lucky ones. It was all truly great. I must thank you for keeping that fire alive down through the years. A dear friend you are, Bernd, and ever will be—a great runner to the last.

After quitting sprint speed, I had started distance training, running off the track and up Strawberry Canyon from the UC Berkeley gym, venturing high into the Berkeley hills on a path along a ridgeline of chaparral forest and shrub, then descending Spruce Street back to the gym. Those nearly hour-and-a-half-long runs were perfect midday breaks from my research on the physiology of exercise and body temperature regulation of bumblebees, where I was making exhilarating physiological discoveries in the lab, supplemented by behavioral ones in the field while home in Maine during the summers. This work resulted in my book *Bumblebee Economics*, which twice garnered nominations for the National Book Award in science and earned invitations to write several op-ed pieces for the *New York Times*.

The biologist and naturalist E. O. Wilson invited me to spend a year at the Museum of Comparative Zoology at Harvard, where he confided to me the ambition he had once had to be a runner, as he had apparently noticed my daily run from the museum to Fresh Pond and back. We discussed our relative running expertise, and he was bold enough to tell me that he thought I might be able to run a sub-2:30 marathon. So I credit him with sparking my idea of reaching that goal.

The official marathon distance of 26.2 miles seems odd, but it is, like all the other distances run competitively, enshrined by and retained in history. I also associate the marathon with the marble statue of the *Winged Victory of Samothrace* (also called the *Winged Nike*), a replica of which stood on the grave of my father's sister in Poland, who died during the 1918–19 influenza pandemic while nursing her ill fiancé, who lived. It was put there by her mother, my paternal grandmother, an artist of nature who had studied in Paris. The Nike on that grave is based on the original that is now in the Louvre and was created in the second century BC by a Greek sculptor. I wondered if it might have been associated with the famous run of the soldier Pheidippides to proclaim ""Nikomen!" (We win!) in the Battle of Marathon, the Greeks' battle with the Persians at the Pass of Thermopylae, in 490 BC. After delivering the news of victory, Pheidippides was said to have collapsed and died. The marathon race as such was first run in the 1896 Olympics in Athens, and it seemed that everyone was now running it. I had not dared try it, and it became a challenge to do so and maybe break the 2:30 my friend and biologist colleague had predicted might be possible. Why not try?

Running a marathon would be hard, clean, satisfying, and exciting. In my first one, in San Martin, California, on March 23, 1975, with my Berkeley running buddy Peter Day, we finished together in a tie in 2:35. We had tested the waters and all seemed fine as we had kept a good pace to the end, so it seemed safe to start faster the next time, which was for me the Boston Marathon a month later, where I ran fifteen minutes faster. I gave it another go four and a half years later, on October 28, 1979, in the Golden Gate Marathon in San Francisco.

The *San Francisco Examiner*'s Monday, October 29, headline read "Complete Unknown Wins Marathon." "In that race," the story ran, "a 22-year-old local, Peter Demaris, took the lead ahead of the 1,100 runners. He kept increasing his lead until he was a full half mile ahead at 20 miles into the 26.2-mile race." The piece then continued:

> The guy in second place was some ancient 39-year-old whom no one had ever heard of. He'd only run two marathons, and that was five years ago. He had never run this course, and in this race, he was far behind the youthful Demaris on the hilly route, running into headwinds. Waiting at the finish, the race announcer received a message from the last route checkpoint and told the crowd that Peter Demaris had a huge lead and should arrive in ten minutes. Ten minutes later, "Here he comes!" he shouted, and the crowd started cheering, "Here he is, the winner—number 1329, Bernd Heinrich."

I now have only one memory of that marathon of more than forty years ago. I recall the last half minute, when I was coming around a bend in an alley, a wall of people on both sides, seeing the finish line up ahead with a runner nearing it. I thought I might be able to catch him, so I sprinted, caught up, and passed him at the finish by perhaps a foot or two. I was disappointed by my time of 2:29:16, having that week run 97 miles in training for the race. But I had entered the race as an afterthought, considered the race itself to be merely a training run, and the next day ran 11 miles. I finished the week with 117 miles, and the next with 143.

The Golden Gate Marathon was not meant to be my real effort; that would be a race four months later, the West Valley Marathon in San Mateo, California. That time I shaved my time down to 2:22:35, coming within 41 seconds of the qualifying time of 2:21:54 to compete in the Olympic trials. It was, however, 1980, the year the Olympics were boycotted by the United States and many other countries. The race did, however, have one consolation: it qualified me to run again in the Boston Marathon only two months later, on April 21, two days after my fortieth birthday. I would be competing in an age category then considered that of "old age" runners. It was then indeed a race against the clock, no longer one with *the* best runners.

Having qualified to run in the Boston Marathon, I was very happy to be home in Maine early, in April, when the willows were in bloom, the woodcock sky-danced, and the bumblebee queens were coming out of hibernation, emerging from the ground. I spent a week before the race on the farm setting out six-inch-square boxes filled with soft, fluffy material to attract the queens to build their nests in. An overwintered queen that I hoped would find one of the boxes would bring in pollen to make a big clump, lay about a dozen eggs into it, then incubate the eggs as a bird does. She would shiver to produce heat with her flight muscles and shunt the heat from them into her smooth abdomen, pressed onto the nest contents, as I had found out in the lab at UC Berkeley and published in the British journal *Nature*. She would then hatch her first clutch of daughters (males are produced only in the fall), and I would later mark the young bee workers with numbered and uniquely colored tags so I could follow their individual foraging careers through the coming summer, when I would literally chase behind them to trace their foraging routes among the various plants that came into bloom throughout the season.

A year before running the upcoming marathon, I had published a research paper in *Science* titled "Keeping a Cool Head: Thermoregulation in Honeybees," and a week before the marathon had talked about this bee thermoregulation physiology with my students in my UC Berkeley comparative physiology lecture, pointing out that my friend Jack Fultz had four years previously likely been able to win the 1976 Boston Marathon on one of the hottest days in history by repeatedly dousing his head with water from a squeeze bottle. I subsequently discovered that bees, when I overheated them, effectively do the same thing to cool down to be able to keep on flying. But not having a squirt bottle, they do it instead by regurgitating liquid from their honey-stomach, the tank they otherwise use to ferry nectar and water into the hive.

The Boston Marathon had loomed as a worthy event to me, because at age forty it seemed like a climax, where I would try my best and then be done with running for good, having done my best To fire myself up, I suffused my brain with the thunderous beat and searing words of Cat Stevens's "Bitterblue." Yes, I'd "been running a long time—eons been and gone—I gave my last chance to you—I've done all one man can do—don't pass me up" I had imbibed the words to be able to recite them in my head throughout the race, to keep up the energy, staying with the rhythm and the beat.

The dense crowd of us packed onto the street in Hopkinton started to creep forward after we heard the starter's gun somewhere in front of what looked like more than a thousand people. I shuffled forward into the fray, and the music went silent. I remember passing a lot of runners, and then reaching so-called Heartbreak Hill. It didn't live up to its reputation because I was by then doing more passing than before, including of a runner crumpled along the sidelines. I heard someone say they thought he was a recent Boston Marathon winner and a world-class Olympian from Canada.

He had probably become dehydrated or had started out too fast and had not been cooling himself with enough water. It had been another hot and muggy day, and I was slipping in my running shoes from the water sprayed on the runners by helpful spectators along the way.

Bill Rodgers won the men's race in 2:12:11 and said it was his toughest ever, but his greatest satisfaction was that he had felt like quitting but didn't. Toshihiko Seko of Japan was second. I won the Masters division in 2:25:25, and it came with a monstrous trophy. I had long forgotten about that trophy until Max, reminiscing about the Berkeley days, told me, "I recall the trophy vividly. We had brought 5 or 6 of your running buddies to your home in Walnut Creek where you showed it to us. It stood on the floor of your living room like a sculpture. It was utterly impressive and must have been 4 feet tall."

I have saved the small metal inscription from it, which says it all, and that is enough.

9

Running After Dreams

IT IS HARD TO KNOW WHERE THINGS WILL LEAD IF YOU GO
with the flow. At age forty, the runners' biological clock says we're
heading "over the hill." And that can make you wonder whether
to keep on running or to give it a rest when you can't give it your
best. Running at one's best is hard, but it is necessary to feel that
difficulty to earn rewards. So you can, of course, keep on running hard until the day you die, but if you've run your best so
far, there is hardly a chance that you'll ever be able to run faster
or farther.

My day of reckoning had already arrived, I suspected, about
a decade or two earlier, maybe near when I had run my first Boston Marathon. However, at the venerable age of forty I was still
running well, and if the endings of the last two races were an
indication, I would have done even better than well if the races
had been longer than the marathon. A small voice grew louder
in my brain the more I thought about it. It said simply, "Run a
longer race—try the 50k."

That summer our family moved from the San Francisco Bay
Area to Burlington, Vermont, where I took a position in the Biol-
ogy Department at the University of Vermont. There in the winter
I resumed cross-country skiing but soon found a local running

community, did some road racing, and then even planned to run in a 50k race coming up in September in Brattleboro. But at almost the last moment on the morning of the race I started wondering if it was worth it. 50k? Really? Why? I had broken the two-minute half mile, I had won a marathon . . . What more? Hadn't that been enough? The thought of getting up before daylight and making the long drive to run nearly defeated me. But Kitty shamed me and practically kicked me out of bed: "*No!*" she said emphatically. "You have to go." Okay. And so we went. It was a close call but a good one, as it turned out.

To my surprise I was passing runners in the last two miles and finished third in 3:03:56. But this time it was not just any runners I passed. One was Frank Bozanich, the open (any age) US record holder of the premier ultrarunning distance, the 100k. I had outraced him in the last miles after he had, I heard, "just spent the summer racing in Europe." He was known as the best. There was now a new ray of light, the possible improvement rather than decrement of running performance; it was at least theoretically possible to set a US record!

I could easily excuse myself for not winning but not for not trying to do what was both worthy and possible. Yet my biological clock was now ticking almost loudly in my brain—I would have to try *now*, as I had already passed my fortieth birthday and there would not be another chance. Not in this life. Do it, or forever regret it, I told myself, so I had to. The race to try would be in a year at the US National Championships, to be held on October 4 in Chicago.

There was not much time left over for running amid my full teaching and research schedule at the university. But to race such a long distance required training more than an hour each day. My only excuse for thinking of competing was that though it would not be my last time running, it would be my last race ever, so it had better be a good one. Achieving the goal would be possible only if everything went right, and that required convincing myself that it was important enough to run at least ten miles a day and sometimes twenty, maybe even thirty, for at least two months.

The only time such a time investment would be possible would be the next summer, when I would be free from my academic duties but could continue my ongoing fieldwork in nearby Maine, where I had, while still in California, purchased a piece of land with a one-room tar paper–covered hunting shack deep in the woods, high on a hill near my hometown. It was without electricity or water but with a weathered sign reading "Kamp Kaflunk" nailed over a recycled door with flaking white paint. It was tucked into a forest of spruce, fir pine, and maple, with the scattered fields of a long-abandoned farm overgrown with shrubs and goldenrods nearby. There were tamarack- and black spruce–rimmed bogs and blueberry bush–covered mountains within running distance, and the spot had for several years been my summer haunt and ecological research area for bumblebees. But I had then stayed at my parents' nearby farm. With Kamp Kaflunk as my new headquarters, Kitty gone back to her home state of California, and Maggie Eppstein as my new wife, we realized that as a modern couple we needed an upgrade from the tar-paper shack.

It may be hard to believe, and it is even harder for me to admit that to be sufficiently motivated to get out of bed that morning the previous year and then drive to Brattleboro to run in the 50k, the opinion of my beloved partner Kitty had been enough. But to do that every day for several months of training in order to race a 100k in Chicago, something truly challenging, would require more than pride; it had to be something greater than the personal. I then recalled as a kid at the Adams farm seeing the image of a man named Ted Williams plastered on a Wheaties box. Why was he the chosen one who, it was believed, would make people eat Wheaties? It was because he was "a great hitter." Then I thought, if I win this thing, I might be considered a great runner, and who wouldn't rather be a runner than a hitter? And if people will eat Wheaties because a great hitter does, maybe they will love and protect Nature more if a great runner does, too. I knew I could not divulge such egotistical irrationality to anyone or it would lose its motivational power. It was to be kept a secret, maybe forever. Luckily, Maggie agreed to join me that summer at Kamp Kaflunk, our tar-paper shack, in a happy and free-running multi-species association of Bubo, a great horned owl, two young crows, and Bunny, Maggie's yellow cat. I agreed to start creating a residence upgrade, building a new cabin, this one out of logs from the surrounding woods. I then sharpened my ax and started felling, delimbing, and debarking spruce and balsam fir trees, something I had not done since a symbolic start in the woods as a young teen at Good Will; here I would continue to completion.

But then within days the world changed and the dream seemed over: somehow I slipped, twisting my leg and breaking the medial meniscus of one knee. I knew what it was immediately, because I had experienced the same accident years earlier in the other knee after trying to push-start my stalled car in the Sugarloaf ski area parking lot. This time I immediately went to the hospital to plead for an operation *now*, on the grounds that I needed it to run a 100k race in the fall. Dr. Helmut Bitterauf, the resident surgeon and a friend, performed the operation within a day, and I resumed running in two weeks. The accident and operation constituted another disadvantage besides my age, adding more challenge to the venture.

The Chicago race was two races in one; runners could finish at the 50k mark or continue on to the 100k. I ran both races, running through the 50k mark, continuing to the finish at the 100k, and finishing in 6:38:21. I did not know what it meant at the time, because I had told myself that after having made the decision to do my best, practical concern for the outcome would no longer be required. It was only long after the race that I learned I had set four records: the any-age US record for 100k, the over-forty world and US records at 50k, and the overall world record at any age for that distance run on the road (which, as I write this thirty-nine years later, has since been bested by 10 minutes and 37 seconds by Max King).

No, I did not get an offer to do a Wheaties ad. By the time I finished the 100k race, the reporters had left, having all focused on the known star ultrarunners, including Barney Klecker, the world record holder of the 50k, and his well-known challengers, in the anticipated battle for first place that had been highlighted at the news conference the night before. The anticipated front-runners had all been spent in their epic battle by the time they reached the 50k mark, while I was far behind them, as a complete unknown. There was no reason for the reporters to hang around, and with the multiple loops to be run, there was no way for casual spectators to know who was where, unless one was focusing on a specific runner. But it was the most satisfying race of my life so far. It reminded me that we can become more than we think ourselves capable of becoming. We are closer to the antelope and to other animals than we think and can even be compared to an ant.

A friend and physiological ecologist colleague, Professor

Rüdiger Wehner at the University of Zurich in Switzerland, compared my performance to that of the African desert ant, *Cataglyphis fortis*. This animal is a fast runner, and like us it evolved as a predator and scavenger in a searing-hot desert environment. Perhaps like us several millions of years or so back, the ant relied on carcasses for its food. In this case, though, it is mainly the carcasses of animals killed by the heat rather than those chased down. This ant has, like us, evolved amazing heat tolerance and speed and is thus able to forage over a large area and to then run home after a hunt to a safe, cool subterranean cavity carrying a heat-killed insect. It does not walk, it only runs, and its running speed is enhanced by its body structure, including legs that are longer than those of other ants. Dr. Wehner, using the statistics of my 100k race (2.8 steps per second, step length 1.5 meters) calculated that I had taken about 66,700 steps in 398 minutes and compared that to one of his ants. He wrote me, "As to *Cataglyphis*, in one of the roundtrips [to forage to and from its subterranean nest] we recorded she made nearly as many steps as you made in the 100k run, but at a step-length frequency of 44 steps/second." Those ants are born to run, as we primates are, and for nearly the same reasons.

In *The Lost World of the Kalahari*, the explorer Laurens van der Post poetically described seeing the San (formerly called "Bushmen") run down kudu antelope. The book excited my imagination as I read his descriptions of their racing after antelope with "a reserve of power, and with length and ease of stride, their minds entirely enclosed in the chase and impervious to fatigue." He and a partner followed the runners in a Land Rover, according to their odometer, for about twenty miles, and then "the final mile was an all-out sprint." Van der Post focused on Nxou, one of the runners, who chased down a kudu bull in a herd of about fifty animals. Van der Post concluded, "I am certain they ran as only the Greek who brought the news of Marathon to Athens could have run." Similarly, Elizabeth Marshall Thomas in her book about the same people, *The Old Way: A Story of the First People*, wrote that a man named Short /Kwi once or twice a year might run down an eland. A San husband was expected to hunt, and it was not just for food, because protein was readily available and was often taken from lions and leopards after shooing them off their kills. A main, or at least the immediate, reward of the hunt is mental. The excitement a hunt produces is an ingrained evolutionary stimulus that induces action without the hunter's need of even thinking of a reward, in the same way we get excited about running a race, even when the physical reward of doing so may be no more than a tall piece of fake metal.

10

Cheating the Biological Clock

MY VICTORY IN THE CHICAGO 100K RACE HAD BEEN AGAINST the mechanical clock but also against the largely unseen biological clock in the background. There is honor in cheating this clock. We would like to mock it if possible. None of us can prove it wrong, but everyone hopes to cheat it if they can. It is the avowed enemy of most if not all of us. I had at least symbolically mocked it and could perhaps risk trying to do so once more— although I had promised myself to focus entirely on my research and eventually write a book about the race. But then I had a wild thought: there is another ultra standard, the 100-mile.

Forty miles more than the 100k is a lot, but given my 100k pace and the fact that I had sped up at the end of the race, I might, if I ran at a slower pace, do as well or even better at the longer distance. It might be doable; why not try for the open US 100-mile record?

I could do it, so why *not* do it? Laziness is no excuse. And because of that thought, about four years later, in March 1986, there would be plastered on the front cover of *Running Times* the unreal headline "Ultra-Fast: At Age 45, Bernd Heinrich Is the Best Runner in America at Four Different Distances." In Germany, *Die Zeit* and *Der Spiegel* gave me press coverage as well. The new start came with the Maine Rowdies, a local running club in Brunswick.

The Rowdies were unique, as if from another culture, putting on a forty-eight-hour race on the Bowdoin College 400-meter track, a crazy, unheard-of, nonstandard distance. It made no sense, but they prided themselves on just that, being crazy. They might just go for my idea. I asked their ringleader, Bill Gayton, a professor of psychology at the University of Southern Maine in Portland, "Hey, how about I try for the hundred-mile American record during your two-day event? I should finish in about half a day." He and his crew would already be timing and counting all the laps, so my time could count officially. They were crazy about the idea; they agreed to do it, possibly because they thought just maybe I *could* run a hundred miles and set the US record!

Race day dawned on the Bowdoin College track with a hazy sunrise. The weather forecast could hardly have been worse for ultrarunners: sunshine and predictions of 90-degree temperatures. Heat is a killer when running.

"How are you feeling?" Charles F. Sewall, my brother-in-law, who had agreed to be my handler, asked as we sat at the local McDonald's at 8:30 a.m., getting ready. I had just finished my second order of French toast to fuel up for the planned 100-mile run, and was on my second cup of coffee. Cream, no sugar. I disliked running in the morning. Coffee helped get my metabolism going. In exactly half an hour, the race would begin. The sun was up, and it looked as though the heat wave would continue. Heat kills. It drains your juices. Worse, it draws blood that should be supplying nutrients to your muscles to your skin instead. I felt disappointed and a bit scared. Would my training go down the tubes?

I had come to run a record and felt ready to give it an honest try, but if I were to have any chance of success in setting the 100-mile record, then every little thing had to be perfect. It wasn't. What now? Go home? No! I had too much mental and physical training invested. Then it occurred to me that the nights were cooler than the days, and if I ran *another* standard ultra-race instead, the twenty-four-hour race for distance, I would be heat-hampered for only half the time: I would be running at a slower pace in the day, but in running at night half of the time, I might still be able to make the longer-distance record, the other golden ultra-distance mark, the standard twenty-four-hour run. The chances were slim but the margin better. And so there on the spot, we switched the target from the 100-mile run to the twenty-four-hour challenge.

"Great!" I said. "Let's go!"

The spur-of-the-moment switch from the anticipated half-day race to an all-day-and-night one was not easily done, but neither had been the preparation for it. In the preceding week it had involved two days of carbohydrate depletion by running to exhaustion while empty, followed by two days of carbohydrate loading (this then-standard practice has now been deemed use-less), timing it all so that the last poop would be out shortly before the start of the race. I had never before conceived of running all day and all night, but our decision was quick enough not to engage much thought or arouse much concern. And then it was time, as twenty or so of us runners lined up on the track and heard "On your mark, get set—go!"

Once we started, things went smoothly and all seemed okay. The hours flew by.

I sometimes mentally blanked out of the fray, visualizing pleasant things or trying to go on automatic. And then there were times when I tried to fine-tune the "machine" so it would run on autopilot by taking time to think about the rhythm of the legs and the breathing, and engaging deliberate mental concentration to relax for smoothness in stride.

The idea is to be aware of every movement so that you can feel the rhythm well enough to control it. Take hip movements: with each stride, the hip of the leading leg shifts slightly forward just as the foot strikes the ground and the same-side arm swings in the opposite direction and acts as a counterweight.

Normally, I'm not at all consciously aware of where my right arm and right hip are when my right foot swings forward and where they are when it swings back. But after monitoring a few dozen strides, I begin to have a conscious awareness of how each part moves relative to the others. Now I could control them. That might lead to a slightly loping stride; now I have corrected and adjusted that side so it feels just right, and I relax my mind in stages and let it run on automatic while doing the same on the other side. And voilà, eventually I can have both sides simultaneously in my mind. Suddenly I feel smooth and in control, an economical smoothness. Then I go back to dreaming . . . lap after endless lap. In the afternoon, after I'd reached ninety miles, a friend, fellow runner, and biologist colleague F. Daniel Vogt stopped by for a visit. He handed me a cup of warm coffee, a welcome reprieve from the baby food that Charlie was handing me after I requested it every few miles for fuel, when I had the appetite.

Soon it was night and eerily quiet. Charlie got drowsy and slumped into his seat by the track, missing a few laps during which I might have wanted water or food. The nighttime hours went on forever, and rather than staying on full alert I tried at times to relax, by snap-sleep moments of closing my eyes for a few seconds, but only on the straightaways. It is easy to step off the track on the curves. After having an intense desire to see the dawn I finally did—and I will never forget hearing the first crows' calls. The sun would soon be rising, and then it would only be a few more hours!

Then the sun did come up bright and clear, and it quickly got hot. Some of the contestants started walking. Some took naps. One was taken to the hospital. I tried some more sleep running, negotiating sections of the straightaways with my eyes closed. A fellow runner wore a black eye patch instead. Whether he knew it or not, he was using a tactic some birds and dolphins do; they switch their sleep from one side of the brain to the other and thus can keep going while half awake on transoceanic migrations or, in the case of dolphins, while swimming.

For me the race would end at exactly the same time it started the previous day, to the second. Since I was running faster than anyone else, and since the race director knew the score, the track gossip was that I was going for the US twenty-four-hour record. I could sense a mounting excitement. Calculations were made, and I was informed that I had a chance but "you need to pick it up just a little." *Oh my God, oh my God*, I was thinking. I *have* to do it. It is within reach, and it can all be decided by mere yards, theoretically just one yard. The bystanders wanted to see me make it almost as much as and perhaps even more than I did. I knew they did; they were runners, too, and I felt them running with me in spirit. I could not disappoint them. They knew exactly what was happening in my mind and body. I had so much invested in this race, so much to gain, so much to lose—if I missed this magical distance mark (I did not know what it was) by just one yard, it would not be a record and all my hard work would have been for nothing. That was what made it great. Hang in, I told myself. One lap. Run this one lap. That's all there is right now. Nothing else. This lap. Now.

There was, finally, I thought, maybe only a half hour to go. I was almost there. The air temperature had soared to 90 degrees. I was thirsty. Bill Gayton had set a barrel full of water at the side of the track, and we dunked our heads into it every few laps. It soon smelled gamey. Someone came alongside and handed me a paper cup filled with fresh water. I gulped it down and went on. Darren Billings, a fellow runner who dropped out the night before after ninety miles, came alongside and told me, "It's going to be *close*." He did not say what. The finish? The expected margin? But I knew what he meant: go faster.

Once I knew it would all end soon, I found reserves I couldn't have imagined. My mind had calculated the depletion of my reserves to coincide with the dwindling minutes. Somehow, having run the first fifty miles at an 8-minutes-per-mile pace, I sped up in the last four miles to an average of 7:12 minutes per mile, dipping once into a sub-7-minutes-per-mile pace. I knew the race director would pull a trigger, a pistol shot would sound . . . I would hear it soon . . .

I dropped as though I'd been shot, sprawled flat on the track, lying still until a chalk mark was made and the distance measurements to the last yard taken. I lay still until race officials dragged me off into the shade under the bleachers and packed me in ice, and then I began to shake violently. That symptom seemed alarming, and race director Gayton ordered an ambulance. I heard the siren coming. They lifted me onto a stretcher, and the next thing I knew, I was in a comfy bed in a Portland hospital, saline dripping into a vein. A priest came into my empty room and was standing over me with a few words to say. But I was smiling; I was already recovering. I had not been ill. Rehydration, rest, and now the warm bed had done magic. I had never felt more wonderful. I had been dehydrated and had merely been in heat prostration. Had they just left me to lie in the shade for a few minutes with a glass of water, instead of packing me in ice, I'd have been fine in five minutes.

My body had been doing everything it could to get rid of its built-up heat, and it had done a great job of it but had been running low on water as I had not stopped to drink during the last few miles. But then, the instant after the *Bang!*, the massive internal heat production, coupled with the huge heat input from the sun, had stopped while my whole body was at the same time bathed in ice. My body temperature would have plummeted instantly, and the temperature control mechanism of the brain would then have suddenly reversed its orders from enabling gradual heat loss by peripheral blood flow to instigate violent shivering for heat production and peripheral blood reduction. Now, in the hospital bed, I was fully awake, and for the rest of the day I felt as if the previous pain, and even the day, had not existed. I was not sleepy. I simply felt as if a day had been deleted.

My mind's aim in running had for months been to achieve the 100-mile record. Instead, when asked for it, the forty-three-year-old body had set the US open twenty-four-hour record, achieving 156 miles and 1,388 yards. Without my knowing it until much later, it had also along the way set the any-age American record for 200k in 18:30:10. The running pundit Stan Wagon declared the run "truly extraordinary" in *UltraRunning* and voted it the "Top Male Performance" of 1983, but not until an objection had to be cleared; my running speed in the last few miles had been unprecedented, and the judges to whom the records were submitted for certification deemed it to have been impossible without some kind of aid.

Little did I know at the time that because of this race and specifically because of Darren Billings's running in it, there would arise from it an opportunity to run in a 100-mile race for a US open record after all, and along with that an opportunity to do some of my most satisfying scientific work on insect body temperature regulation physiology. I could not quit now.

Thermal physiology, especially as applied to endurance, is

hugely important in animal exercise. After my studies at UCLA on sphinx moths, I had gone on to study winter-flying owlet (noctuid) moths in Vermont and Maine. Because these moths are midgets in comparison to most sphinx moths, they necessarily lose heat fast and passively while at the same time being forced to be active in icy-cold weather, perhaps as an evolutionary strategy to escape their bird predators. They are thus limited in their ability to fly by their insufficiently high body temperature. They are like us if we were naked and had to escape polar bears by running in an arctic winter.

Darren was a member of the Maine Rowdies running club, which had organized the race at Bowdoin. He worked as a lab technician in the US Army labs at Natick, Massachusetts, designing and testing clothing for soldiers in various climatic conditions, presumably including the Arctic. One of the tools the army used was thermovision cameras, which sense heat, to discern by color the locations where heat might leak from different kinds of clothing worn in arctic conditions. In my research on insect physiology, I deduced that winter-flying owlet moths are aided by some apparent magic to reduce heat loss to various body parts, especially to the head and abdomen. But my fine "thermometers" (thermocouples) were too large to get accurate measurements of anything that small, since the probe itself would withdraw heat and reduce the subject's temperature. A thermovision camera, which registers temperature in photos without contacting the subject, would be key to getting the data.

Darren had cheered me on in the twenty-four-hour race and at the US Army Research Laboratory, and he had access to thermovision equipment that I could never afford. It could show in color precisely where and how much heat is lost from a person's body, and I thought it might also be able to provide the same information for moths. He offered to set me up to get the data I wanted on moths, on the condition that I run on the lab's treadmill for some tests of human physiology. Fair trade. I went.

We got gorgeous pictures of winter moth temperatures with colors from blue to red showing precisely what I needed to know. I then published a paper in *Science*, which ran a color photo on the cover of the moths' equivalent of a fur coat. Most of the work was expanded in the *Journal of Experimental Biology* and later also featured in *Scientific American*. In turn, Darren's data of my running on the lab's treadmill were published in a paper in *UltraRunning*.

And then the kicker: given the lab results of me on the treadmill, Darren thought I could, despite my advanced age, still set the US record in the 100-mile run, and to support his data he needed to test this hypothesis. I owed him and myself, and he volunteered to drive me to Ottawa, Ontario, where the international running club Sri Chinmoy was putting on a twenty-four-hour track race. I had, of course, absolutely no motivation to run another twenty-four-hour race, but could now finally try for the US open 100-mile record that both Darren and I thought was possible.

How could I not? When fate drops something into your lap, you grab it. And so, at the age of forty-four, I went to Montreal, and lo and behold, I set the US open 100-mile record in 12:27:02, close to the time Darren had predicted for me. I remember little of the run except that I did not make one stop or walk a step along the way, and as I passed one runner on the quarter-mile track a second time, he sang to me, "It's a long way to Tipperary, it's a long way to go." Maybe he thought I was running the twenty-four-hour race and would burn out. I remember no more of the event except that a smiling bald man came up to me to congratulate me after I had stopped at 100 miles. As I learned a little later, it had been the great Sri Chinmoy himself, the international mystic and world peace leader who preached transcendence through running with the messages "Run to become," "Become to achieve," and "Daring enthusiasm and abiding cheerfulness can accomplish anything on earth without fail."

Minutes after the race that afternoon, I was very cheerful as I relaxed on the bleachers watching the twenty-four-hour racers continue, not yet knowing but soon learning who the man was whom I had just met, and that he was a vegetarian. I was then ravenously consuming a great big juicy post-race steak that Darren had thoughtfully provided. He had brought it, no doubt, in remembrance of its appeal at some previous post–Rowdies race party. I do not recall if it was during the one where I had fueled up during the race only with beer or the one where I had fueled up with chocolate ice cream. I felt that one would be better than the other, but which one would depend on the race conditions. I hadn't seen any prior data, so I wanted to find out for myself. With ice cream I won and set a record; with beer I dropped out somewhat short of the finish. Numerous trials might be needed to sort that out, but I suspect beer might win over ice cream on a hot day. The steak was not for fuel but for rebuilding damaged muscle. I noticed that on long runs I smelled of urea, a by-product of protein breakdown that excretes the nitrogen from it and is released in sweat; though I had not been eating protein during the run, I might have been burning body protein for fuel.

One year later, I took advantage of my increasing age to compete in my first race in the venerable forty-five-and-over category. It was again on the track in Brunswick, at another Maine Rowdies event, and this time I was trying to set the over-forty age records for both the fifty miles and 50k on the track. But the surprise added bonus was even better: I set the US open any-age record for 100k on the track in a time of 7:00:12.

11

On the Road to Sparta

BY 1985, I HAD SET SO MANY OPEN ULTRARUNNING RECORDS THAT IN his annual review in *Ultrarunning* magazine, Nick Marshall described me as "the finest American ultra-marathoner of this era." It was a high accolade to live up to, but it had never been my agenda to try. I was then a professor of biology at the University of Vermont, and that demanded sustained and detailed attention to my students. But even more, I was deeply involved with ravens, as a consequence of my familiarity with bees and their social behavior and long fondness of crows and ravens as friends and companions. Given this context, I stumbled onto a gripping question on their, and perhaps general, social behavior. As in running, the research itself was a social undertaking. At an event we held, called "Raven Roundups," we built giant aviaries in the forest at the camp Maggie and I had previously built in the Maine woods. It was a party with hundreds of volunteers who worked for free to produce a fun event, fueled by beer and a pig roasting over a firepit. Marshall listed ten of the most notable ultramarathoners of that year, and not surprisingly the "most notable, Bernd Heinrich," he wrote, "drew a blank." It was not because I hadn't been physically active. I had run another 100k with the Maine Rowdies on the track, finishing in 7:00:11, but more significantly, the famous "Spartathlon" race in Athens a month later. My overall prior main exercise had arguably been dragging animal carcasses through the woods, although afterward that often required me to sit still for hours in the snow hidden under fir branches, and/or climbing to the tops of spruce trees for views into the distance to keep track of my birds. But being invited, all expenses paid, to run the prestigious 245-kilometer (152-mile) Spartathlon from Athens to Sparta was an experience that seemed worth going out of the way for, a once-in-a-lifetime opportunity.

I had started running in February after returning from East Africa on a research trip with my student Brent Ybarrando to celebrate his PhD thesis accomplishment of a study on the physiology of diving by water beetles. I would take him to study dung beetles' thermal physiology in South Africa, a follow-up from my years-earlier experiences with elephant dung beetles in Tanzania and then Kenya. To again study those chunky, almost bird-sized insects, Brent and I had to be among elephants producing dung, in areas where it was also prudent to be cautious of lions. Running was not on the agenda. However, after returning to Vermont, I ran an average twenty to thirty miles most weeks of February, March, and April. By the end of May, I had then increased to seventy-five miles per week, having by then also traveled to Utqiagvik (formerly Barrow), Alaska, for a week of research on bumblebees' adaptations to that high arctic environment. There, at the research station along the coast, I had not run, due to the presence of polar bears, except for a very unlikely and unanticipated one-mile race. As bizarre as it may sound, that race was of, for, and against—you won't believe it—Frank Bozanich, the very man who had given me the inspiration to race the clock to challenge his American 100k record. I had no clue where he had been in all those intervening years.

At the time, Utqiagvik was still called Barrow. It is a tiny Inuit village at the northern edge of Alaska directly on the shore of
the Arctic Ocean. I would have stood out there among the Inuit,
and Frank, employed as a policeman there, had either noticed
me or had been alerted to my presence. We met and were both
hugely surprised, having had no contact whatsoever in the last
five years after we had raced in the 50k US Championship race
in Brattleboro that had been the impetus for me to become an
ultramarathoner. It was just about the least likely place possible
to meet again, and he seized the opportunity to challenge me to
a one-mile race, one that quickly grew to include a squadron of
local Inuit. At the appointed time we all lined up along the shore
of the Arctic Ocean, and right from the start Frank sprinted to
the lead, and stayed there the whole way.

After Alaska, at my camp in Maine back with the ravens, I
penned the following in my log, which I titled "The First Run."
It was a jaunt of some consequence for its distance, and it reads:

Up to 21 June I have been fooling around. For a month I
have run 40–75 miles a week. I have even run a couple of
18 milers, and they didn't go badly. This is all part of the
feeling-out process. Am I still the man who ran 156.8 miles
in 24 hours? I'm still intimidated by that—and at the same
time confident. I'm not sure which. Well, this week I started
working out. Sunday I put in 14 miles, Tuesday 15, and this
morning 21. Now in the afternoon cool drizzle at 8:00 a.m.
is the perfect time to really put the hammer down, to run my
20-mile loop around Lake Webb to see what I'm still made
of. And already at the 10-mile mark I knew there would be
trouble—I was 16 minutes off my best time for the corner by
the Carthage pizza. And then I really started to fade. Slowly,

inexorably, each step got weaker. I felt dizzy and could barely lift my legs. That was at barely 15 miles—not even halfway through. I needed food. I was hypoglycemic—even though my sense of needing food was an insignificant cry for the need to stop. Only my brain, my reason, told me, "if you want to keep lifting those legs, you've got to get something into your stomach." So I stopped at the nearest farmhouse. "Have you got a cookie, piece of bread, anything?" I asked the woman who came to the door to my knocking. She did have a piece of white bread but said "I don't have any cookies." I gulped the piece of mushy bread like a ravenous wolf, and on I went. Slowly, I could again lift my legs. Until I made it to the Weld store, where I got (on credit) 2 bottles of juice, a Milky Way candy bar, and a banana, from Gerry, the storekeeper. At that time, I was in a delirious state again and could not lift my legs. But after this snack I was off jogging again and made it back up the mile-long hill to the cabin—to fall exhausted into a deep sleep on my bed, without even taking my shoes off. So much for my first workout. 20 miles in 3:03. Do I have the courage to endure this twice per week for four months [my intended run of a race on September 27 in Greece] with no assurance that I'll be healthy on the day of the race, and otherwise lose it all? Getting ready to climb Mt. Everest would be preferable, and easier.

I then went back to Vermont and logged 173 miles in July, 485 miles in August (which included the Rowdies' 100k that I did in racing speed), and 130 miles the week before the race in Greece. I felt prepared, and once in Athens, the day before the Spartathlon start, I met my friend and fellow runner of previous races Ray "the K" Krolewicz from Columbia, South Carolina, who would also be racing the next day. He said, "Bernd, you could win this race!" His comment made me nervous. I have high expectations of myself, but others' having them for me is different. I ran several laps on a nearby 400-meter track to try to loosen up for the race the next morning.

We started the race literally in the pitch dark of what seemed night in what looked like a street in any other town, and this was what I wrote afterward:

> We gather in predawn darkness on the outskirts of Athens, waiting for the bus to take us to the Olympic Stadium at the city center. The air is still, and there are only occasional hushed murmurings among us athletes from different countries. We are supposedly among the best in the world, and I feel greatly honored and touched to have been one of the few chosen to represent the U.S.A. It still seems like a dream. I had only seen pictures of the ancient stadium where the Olympics began. But in a little over an hour I would actually see the real thing with my own eyes. And it would be more than a historic monument. It would be the start of a 250 km race.

The Spartathlon commemorates the legend of Pheidippides, a *hemorodromus*, or so-called day runner, used as long-distance messengers over the mountainous Greek terrain. Herodotus mentioned that he was an expert and that the runners were "young men but recently out of their childhood, like those that wear their first downy growth of beard." In other words, maybe a lot like me in high school cross-country: raw and eager.

Pheidippides had left Athens at daybreak on a journey that included mountainous terrain with a downhill toward Sparta, for a total distance of about 155 miles (not the 26.2-mile distance it has since shrunk to), and he had completed it in probably forty-one or forty-two hours, whereas present-day expert distance runners such as all the fifteen finishers in the Spartathlon in 1983 finish inside thirty-six hours. Many of us wondered if we would be able to duplicate his run of almost the same distance as my twenty-four-hour run on the level track. The race, which includes a rocky, nearly four-thousand-foot mountain climb as one of its many obstacles, is considered by many people to be the toughest ultramarathon in the world. Most would approach it with a goal of conquering the distance within the thirty-six-hour time limit. But I did not consider just finishing to be sufficient; my aim was to finish first.

The bus driver wends his way through the morning traffic bravely, as only a Greek driver can (or would). But it could be any big city. Everyone is quiet. We are alone with our private dreams, fears, and aspirations, sealed in by darkness and rumbling traffic as the city wakes. It seems like the calm before a storm. Suddenly we are jolted fully alert as the bus comes to a screeching halt. We look up through the darkness over an acre of marble steps to the hazy outlines of a stone structure: the Olympic Stadium. But it seems anticlimactic now. We will be off in a few minutes and are more concerned with making sure our shoelaces are tied properly. A tiny miscalculation could cost us the race.

We worry about whether or not some other vital detail has been overlooked. The only two women in the race draw reporters like flies. As for the men, three Europeans are picked as the favorites. I do not know any of the runners except Ray; I only get to know their nationalities and associate them with their last names. Ray says again, "This race is made for you, Bernd. You are the dark horse here. You can win it." It is the first (and last) time anyone has said that to me.

Ray is wishing me well. We two do not consider ourselves competitors. The distance and the time are our opponents. The "have to" mind-set has now added to my anxiety, but I try to brush it aside and relax. To win and to go for the highest award takes confidence in oneself that one has done the training and has the skills and tools to maximize one's chances. Then it takes grit and resilience and pure drive and action. When the going gets tough and someone passes me, I will have to remain convinced that I am better than he is. Otherwise, I may be unwilling to try to dig up my reserves to make a comeback. Talent can allow me to become good, but to excel in a crisis will require pigheadedness, blind obstinacy, and maybe even an inflated opinion of my ability. But I'm doing it for myself, not because anybody wants me to. Indeed, these may be the most crucial elements. However, confidence that is too great reduces effort where it counts even more: during the months of training and at the beginning of the race, where caution is just as essential. The former is long past. All I now see is the race looming ahead like a threatening monster.

At ten miles, a group of us are relaxed and appreciating the girls along the sidewalks, waving back at the honking truck drivers, smiling at the clapping bystanders, all the while feeling light-footed, as if we could run forever. The pace seems agonizingly slow; the only question is, am I holding back enough? Although I usually run alone, today I enjoy the company of others. Along freeways, past Coca-Cola signs, eucalyptus trees, and red hammer-and-sickle slogans spray-painted on walls, the Hungarian and I are now alone together, looking straight ahead. We are already hot and keep changing the lead, helping break the stiff headwind for each other.

At first, my steps were effortless and unnoticed. Now I am becoming conscious of them, the endless *slap, slap, slap* of rubber on pavement, the same monotonous rhythm hour after hour. Some five hours into the run, we have left the outskirts of Athens far behind. Winding roads hug the rugged coastline, and the chaparral reminds me of California. It could be Highway 1 north of San Francisco. It is dry and windy, and the bright sun is starting to burn. Ernő Kis-Király, the Hungarian, is a superb marathoner. He is keeping up the pressure, but we are running like a matched team. When I try to hold back a little, he turns and slows, asking in shrugs and upturned palms if I feel okay. Him asking *me* if I feel okay! I come alongside again, his gestures having given me a flash of doubt: Maybe I won't pick him off so soon after all. Am I getting weaker, or is it these steep hills? The Hungarian's coach leans out of a car and shouts instructions. Kis-Király shrugs and speeds up ever so slightly. I follow along. The rhythm of the miles returns me to a song by Cat Stevens: "Summer's come and gone / Drifting under the dream clouds / Past the broken sun." Dream clouds indeed. I'm under the spell. My companion has become a friend. He gestures with the fingers on one hand to indicate how many runners are still ahead, and I smile and gesture back by pulling on a make-believe rope, to tell him we'll soon be reeling them in. He smiles his understanding under his long black mustache. On a long open stretch, we glimpse two runners ahead of us. We'll soon overtake them. Kis-Király looks like a well-oiled machine. His slender legs pump rhythmically, and his thick chest heaves just barely. Determination shows in his eyes under his mane of flying black hair. Perhaps, like me, he is wondering how Pheidippides felt as he was running, knowing the people of Athens were waiting for the news of their fate and that delivering it depended on his legs.

After a few more curves we come up to the Dane Mogens Feld, who has run sixty-two marathons with a best time of 2:16. I looked him over as a possible threat before the start. He stays with us for a few miles; then we cruise past him. As with so many others he sinks from sight, as I expect for a mere marathon runner. I expect Kis-Király to do the same, soon. At fifty miles, only Dusan Mravlje the Yugoslav is still in front of us.

It seems as though we've been running a long time, but I now realize with a shock that the race has barely begun and already I'm beginning to have to work to keep up with the Hungarian. Is he losing his head trying to catch the leader? I let him go and follow the Spartathlon signs deeper into the hinterlands alone. There are gravelly tracks through vineyards laden with ripe grapes, where wizened old farmers ride on creeping donkey carts. The little towns at intervals are invariably populated by swarms of kids running out to greet me, as they do for all the runners. They jog or ride their bicycles alongside me shouting: "American? American?" One presses a note into my hand. It says, "We love you." Another jogs alongside and hands me a red rose. I carry it for miles, finding it difficult to discard it by the wayside. But suddenly I think of the 4,000-foot mountains that are still ahead and I drop the rose as the prospect looms.

I press on, almost smelling Kis-Király again, and think Mravlje must be around the next turn. The road, now tarred again, snakes up into steep rolling hills through ancient olive groves. My legs start to feel heavy. "Just the hills," I think and keep up the pressure. Then, glancing back down the hill, I see a runner in the distance. That's strange; I knew I had held a huge lead over the next runners. After another turn he is a bit closer. Then he comes alongside. It is Patrick Macke, the British favorite. With a short, smooth stride, he glides effortlessly past me without giving me a sideways glance. I'm in fourth place now, and I have a new sensation: panic! My increasingly difficult labor had not been due to acceleration. I am probably slowing down. Macke is maintaining the same pace he took from step one, independently of any other runners then as now.

Like a barely perceptible irritation that develops over time into a debilitating blister, the bit of excess speed I had forced over the long distance is slowly making its impression. My legs do not lift as easily, and my appetite leaves me. My body, it seems, has enough to do just to keep my legs in motion. I should stop to rest and eat, but my ambition and pain now block and blind my judgment. I cannot conceive of walking and have to fight even harder just to hold my fourth position. If I can only hang on long enough, maybe the others will pull out. Maybe they have overextended themselves. Anything can happen: a pulled muscle, blisters, cramps, hitting a wall.

At eighty miles, I content myself with little goals: making it to the next aid station, over the next rise, past the next curve. But then two unknown runners come up behind me. I have never been passed so far into a race. In the past, I have always done *my* passing then, and all the runners who were passed were invariably passed for good. Another Cat Stevens song returns: "Going round and round / Yes, I've been moving a long time / But only up and down." Visions fly through my mind of other races. I think of the Maine Rowdies' twenty-four-hour race. Although the first seventy-five miles in that run were so relaxed I tried to snooze while running by occasionally closing my eyes, the last six miles were the most painful experience of my life and I reached deep because I promised myself it was a once-in-a-lifetime experience, one never to be repeated. I dulled the pain by concentrating on the smiling faces of my kids, the woods I love, the support of friends, and I accelerated and somehow lived through a few more miles. But then I collapsed, unable to take another step, and paid for it with a day in the hospital. I can try to ignore pain now, but there aren't just six more miles down the road—there are at least seventy.

My legs are stiff, really stiff. Uphill or downhill, it is all the same. Each leg extension is an effort of will. Now Jean-Dominique Calbera, Alfons Everz, Ray Krolewicz, Rune Larsson, and even Mogens Feld will soon be coming up on my heels. I feel them approaching. It seems like a nightmare I used to have where I am running for my life from a fiendish enemy and my legs move sluggishly, as though through cold molasses. With every step I ask myself: What am I doing here and why?

It is almost dark now. The air is chilly, and I'm not burning enough calories to keep warm. My sweaty hair has dried into sticky mats. White rivulets of salt encrust my brow and dangling arms. My head hangs. The law of gravity, it seems, is now the strongest force as I try to walk uphill. Kis-Király has dropped out. Somewhere, miles ahead, Macke is still running strongly.

There is at this point nothing left for me to salvage. I trained hard. There are no promises to keep but miles to go. The time I finish in will make no difference. The only thing that mattered was beating the other runners, and that is not a sufficient reason to go on. An aid station comes into sight. I stop at a table spread with food. Nothing looks appetizing. My overpowering urge is simply to get off my legs. As much to myself as to anyone, I say, "I don't think I can make it." The station attendant responds nonchalantly, "If you drop out, you have to take off your number." That simple? Just take off my number and I can sit down? I inhale deeply. "Okay." It's done. I had not stopped until I'd given everything I had left.

12

Pacing

THE CIRCADIAN CLOCK ENABLES ORGANISMS TO PREPARE themselves to be active at the appropriate times. It acts in flowers to open them at the best time to be pollinated and in bees to fly out and collect the nectar and pollen at the time they are available. Animals become sleepy and/or wakeful at dusk and dawn to initiate their activity, and extreme running requires a choreography of a large number, if not most, of our physiological systems. They cannot all shift into full gear at once. One function after another is activated with respect to time, creating a synchronized system at almost all levels of biology.

In the Spartathlon, the Europeans may have had an advantage over the Americans arriving the day before due to the six-hour time difference, but that would not have explained the difference between me and Ray "The K" Krolewicz. He finished well, and he had seldom been close to me in a race before, even though he had run countless more races than I could ever dream of entering. On the other hand, I was now forty-five and a half years old and may have bumped up against the braking effect of the circannual clock. However, why did I crash at 60 miles when a month earlier I had still been able to run a 100k? Had a month not been long enough for some parts of my system to recover?

Maybe our bodies *do* wear out if we do not allow them enough time to rebuild and recover. Maybe the urea I had smelled was like the smoke of muscle tissue burning because I was not ingesting enough fuel through the digestive tract. Or was it my pacing during the race itself, going out too fast before a critical physiological step had been sufficiently activated? The total energy expenditure of a race would be the same if one started fast and slowed down at the end or started slow and sped up at the end. How had my descent to utter weakness been possible so early in the race? Looking at animals other than ourselves may yield insights.

Alaskan sled dogs, huskies and malamutes, qualify as an example. Running the multiday Iditarod Trail Sled Dog Race of 1,150 miles, they burn more calories per pound of body weight than any other animal species that runs routinely as part of its survival tool kit. The dogs run up to fourteen hours at a time and then, after a few bouts of that, run even more strongly than earlier. It appears that after a certain period of running, their metabolism "flips a switch." How or why they gradually build up their running capacity *throughout the race* rather than slowing down is not known, but a study of the gray tree frog (*Hyla versicolor*), a small tree-climber, suggests a physiological explanation for this endurance phenomenon, one that involves pacing of energy expenditure in their bouts of loud calling.

Tree frogs are best known to physiological ecologists for their ability to prepare for and then survive winter by freezing solid. But in the summer their most important behavior, at least in the males, is a vigorous exercise to attract mates. As the males perch in place, often near many others, they attract the females by advertisement calls that in terms of the volume of the sound they produce is comparable to ours, despite their minuscule body size.

The frog's noise is produced by inflating a balloon-like throat pouch, then forcibly deflating it in a muscle-pumping burst that forces the air over the vocal cords, vibrating them. The more volume a male can achieve, the farther his vocal reach for mates will be, and the more offspring that share his characteristics and capabilities will be produced.

In the natural selection of these loudmouthed frogs, the limiting factor is physical capacity in energy expenditure, not just per individual call but in terms of the ability to keep on making them over long periods of time. In tree frogs this amounts to about 1,400 calls per hour for an all-night performance. The vigor and persistence of the male frogs' nocturnal vocal exercise involve a large portion of their musculature, which may be for us the equivalent of running a marathon and beyond, and it is energetically the most costly activity of any cold-blooded vertebrate. Their display is reserved for the nighttime, because that is the only time the females can abandon their safe hiding spots on tree bark, where they are almost perfectly camouflaged during the daytime and would only be noticed by movement.

The biologists Theodore L. Taigen and Kentwood D. Wells measured the male frogs' energy cost of calling by their rates of oxygen consumption in the lab, although the outcome of the shouting matches with many other males would be inferred to depend on the number of calls a frog could muster per night. The calling rate of any one frog in the chorus increased gradually from about 600 calls per hour at 8:30 p.m. to 1,400 calls per hour a half hour later, at 9:00 p.m. The frogs' whole-body lactate levels (lactate being a by-product of exercise that limits further exercise if it is not removed by sufficient oxygen intake) began to increase as the exercise started but then dropped to half of the previous level as the frogs continued to call and to do so even more frequently. The frogs adjusted metabolically to the increased pace by increasing their calling pace gradually and only to the point where the lactate-burning process was sufficiently activated to remove the increasing amounts of lactate still being produced. Such pacing may apply to our running as well; the human exercise physiologist David Costill, in his book *A Scientific Approach to Distance Running,* showed in a graph that our oxygen uptake during running does not reach a maximum until well into the exercise.

Although the frogs shout while perched in place, this exercise is analogous to our running steps, where achieving the most (in terms of number of calls or steps) requires avoiding lactate buildup by increasing the pace slowly enough to be able to deal with it. A slower initial pace results in more exercise later, as I wrote in an article on the topic for *UltraRunning* magazine titled "The Lessons of the Frogs." But the running theme concerns the physiological limits that have evolved because they were beneficial for survival to and through reproduction.

In frogs, the burden of the exercise of mating falls on the males. The females also become active in the dark of night and travel to find a male, an activity that in terms of energy cost is minor compared to the males' calling. The females are bloated with eggs, but the reproducing males provide only sperm and can each fertilize several females, whereas each female has only one shot at the reproduction lottery per season, and in many species per lifetime. The female is therefore choosier; she goes to where there are the most males to choose from, which is where she hears the most calling coming from. Since that is where the females go, it is also where other males need to go to join the chorus, to make a lot of noise, thus unavoidably facing competition with one another as well as being helped by the amplified volume of the chorus.

It is not only frogs that do this.

One summer on my way through the woods, I saw a gathering of hundreds, maybe thousands, of small animals, all of one kind, gathered in the same place displaying themselves as if in the Boston Marathon, but in this case not moving laterally but vertically. Flies of the family Empididae, like us, are born predators. They were displaying their physical strength, agility, and endurance to prospective mates. Empidid females can be expected to preferentially mate with males that are good or at least persistent flyers, because that is a prerequisite of hunting ability, which determines the ability to leave descendants, which drives evolution. A difference between our lineage and theirs is that they chase their prey on the wing and we hominids do (or did) it by running.

You might wonder why I chose flies as an example. I chose an insect because insects have experienced at least a hundred million years' more time and much more severe elective pressure to evolve than we have, since for every couple hundred young they produce, only one on average survives to reproduce. One could even expect that since we are so much less severely selected at any one time, they may even give us a glimpse of the future with our selection spread over a longer time frame. At least I thought so when comparing their mindless but efficient behavior to ours. If I could not run, I would want to fly, and watching the flies, I could envision it as being fun. It looks as if they are dancing, hence their common name, "dance flies."

Empidid flies' seemingly futile up-and-down "dance" flights are not futile at all. They are like the tree frogs' chorusing groups. They take place in so-called lecks, where males gather to be available for females to come and evaluate and then choose one to mate with. The females' best choice of mate in such a situation would be expected to correlate with health and vigor. Mere flight endurance would matter, since those males that can hang out and stay airborne the longest would increase their chance of mating simply by participating. However, the females have, over time, also evolved to evaluate the males' flight pattern as well. The males would then have experienced selective pressure to sweeten the deal to favor females' choice by offering something aside from their mere presence and perseverance. As predators feeding on other insects, male empidid flies had opportunity to exploit that possibility; in some species males began to bring and carry a prey carcass to the dance that, in addition to the lure of sex, drew a female to the male for the meal he offered. The technique caught on and spread, and then further along the evolutionary progression, the females mated primarily with the males who offered that gift. But with the emphasis gradually shifting to *food* as a means of attraction, some males then used the females' preference and turned it around to their own advantage. As reported by the entomologist Edward L. Kessel for the species *Hilara maura*, the males wrap their prey, bag-like in white silk that stands out visually and also makes the offering *look* larger. The packaging then allowed them to use smaller prey, which led to the evolution of providing less than they advertised simply by more conspicuous packaging, until they stopped putting any prey inside the shiny white silk package at all. The progression is analogous to a beau offering to a woman he's wooing a box of chocolates that, with time and tradition, would be replaced by an increasingly decorated but empty box. I've already been noticing something similar in grocery stores, where there are many beautiful packages of food, but when we get home and open them, we find that they are up to a third to a half empty. The larger-appearing but lightly loaded attraction made the fly dancers lighter, and thus likely more agile and/or longer-enduring dancers than those carrying heavy prey.

We have perhaps not yet individually advanced to this level of sophistication, but that might be debated. One day, upon opening a package of prunes, I noticed in surprise that the colorful carton with pictures of luscious prunes all over it was only half full. It wasn't because it was designed for easy carrying. No; it was designed to look like more than it is. In contrast, blueberries are packed into clear plastic square boxes that show them off. The price of the box was right. But after I had bought it and started eating them, it turned out that the berries were hiding a big hollow; the bottom of the box, instead of being flat, had a hugely bulged-up middle to create empty space in the middle of the berry heap. Okay, it's not for sexual selection, but techniques for changing our appearance in all sorts of ways from the natural, by apparel and paint, are well known. The shoe industry has also been making steady progress when it comes to running, which has been ever more commercialized, to provide massive financial rewards as goads, rewards that enhance sexual and/or mate-finding appeal. (A disclaimer: I have not once received money and/or other material that can be converted to it as a result of my running. But I say, good for them who have. I would have accepted it if offered.)

Material rewards, it needs to be mentioned, will ultimately have consequences, likely unanticipated ones. They did in the dance flies. In the case of *Rhamphomyia longicauda*, an American species, the male gift-giving scenario was upended. Apparently, males in *that* species had been so generous in their gift offerings that the females began to compete among themselves for the males' nuptial gifts. Subsequently, the males became choosier about who they would mate with and began to notice especially those females who advertised themselves the most, which in one species evolved to have prominent pink inflated abdominal sacs. Once the males were the main choosers, the females gathered in groups or swarms and the males flew there to evaluate them and to make their choice.

All that happened, of course, without any individual frog or fly knowing what it was doing or why and what it would lead to. Animals blindly play out programs that are selected for and eventually inscribed in their DNA. At least in the immediate time frame, we know what *we* are doing and why and so can escape purely genetic constraints. Nevertheless, we are unconsciously influenced by and act out innate programs that are reflections of the behavior and physiology of our ancient ancestors. That brings us back to our running, not in terms of a means of feeding ourselves but as a factor in mate selection in our evolutionary past.

Running benefits both males and females because it aids in gathering food and escaping from predators. It became especially useful on the open plains of Africa where, millions of years ago, beginning as poor hunters, we likely scavenged from the kills of large cats and canids. In that cradle of our evolution I had routinely seen vultures spiraling in the sky before descending to a predator-killed carcass, and in the heat of the day seen lions rest in the shade. Because of our ability to sweat, we could run to the scene of a kill indicated by vultures and make use of it for ourselves in the short time during which it is less defended. The more we could tolerate heat and run in it, the more likely we were to run and eat and vice versa and thus be able to feed our offspring. As a result, our sweating response would be selected for all the more. But access to water would have been required.

One difference between us and many other animals (except for many birds) is that our young were not only helpless but also relatively large and not easily transportable; we had no thick hair they could cling to when we moved about. They had instead to be sheltered somewhere, and the female had to be there to nurse them, creating her need for a food provider and therefore needing to base her preference for a mate on the demonstration of his ability and willingness to provide food, as well as a home base. Even up to recent times, in many tribes a male was not allowed to marry until he had proven himself to be a good hunter by providing an eland, a kudu, or some other large prey as proof, options later substituted by perhaps a dinner out, a car, a house, or a big bank account, all indicating the potential to support a family. We are, lock, stock, and clock, biologically the same tribe we have been since long before any history was recorded. We are evolutionarily selected hunters of game.

13

Racing Caterpillars and Exercising Pupae

A WOOLLY BEAR CATERPILLAR WAS HUMPING ALONG OVER A road at a good clip, and I wondered how fast it was running compared to other caterpillars, because why should a caterpillar run at all? Caterpillars feed on leaves, and plants don't run away.

It was September 1994, and over the next several days I picked up caterpillars of other kinds to find out how they compared and wrote the results into a dated notebook. Using my runners' stopwatch, I ended up timing the speeds of thirty-six caterpillars of thirteen species, and to make it fair and even I timed them all on level ground in shade and at temperatures of 70 to 72 degrees F. But other seemingly more urgent things came up, as they usually do, one after another, and for the next twenty-five years I forgot about those caterpillar capers, until recently when I chanced to find the notes in a box of running "stuff" tucked away for possible future use.

Running speed varies widely among different animals, and I had written about the topic relative to bipedalism in *Racing the Antelope*. It turns out that with respect to the number of legs, less is generally more, at least up to a point: a bipedal animal can achieve running speed almost on par with the four-legged world champions, specifically the pronghorn antelope. But in general, the more legs an animal has (and some arthropods, such as centipedes and millipedes, have about fifty and up to two hundred, respectively) the more slowly it moves both in absolute terms and in terms of body lengths per unit of time. Having more legs seems to be the more original, or primitive, condition, with evolution for greater speed and mobility corresponding to loss of legs. Even some fast cockroaches, such as the American cockroach, *Periplaneta americana*, will, when motivated to run fast (as in contests where they are set into the light and scurry off to hide in the dark), run bipedally, leaving their two additional pairs of legs idle and useless. Similarly, one lizard, the basilisk, though normally quadrupedal, will if pressed take off bipedally, moving fast enough to literally run on water, hence its nickname, "Jesus lizard." Caterpillars, however, don't run with their legs. Like imagoes (the "adults" they metamorphose into), they have three pairs of legs, but they are tiny and all at the front end, where they are used for holding and manipulating food. Caterpillars propel themselves not with their legs but with wavelike contractions of the whole body.

My caterpillars would not leave on demand when I set them down. I timed their speed by measuring the distance they covered without stopping after they started on their own and then calculated the time per distance they had moved. Their speed varied enormously from that of one notodontid moth (*Nerice bidentata*), which averaged a slow crawl of 5.8 centimeters per minute, whereas the great tiger moth caterpillar, *Arctia caja*, cruised at 259 centimeters per minute. But my interest was less in their speed, as such, than the differences between species: Why were some caterpillars so incredibly slow and others speed demons more than forty times as fast?

A pattern emerged after I sorted out what differed between

the slow and fast caterpillars. Those that fed on widely dispersed herbs close to the ground raced along at a good clip. On the other hand, those that mimicked leaves or parts of leaves on trees were hard to budge, and when they did, they moved glacially. Those of intermediate speed were species that stayed on the tree or branch where they fed but commuted between nearby feeding and nearby resting or hiding places. The divergence in locomotory speed varying according to feeding habits suggests an advantage for some animals of being almost immobile; speed is related to reaching distant food, as hunters do, or escaping them, as prey does.

Immobility is necessary for some caterpillars' defense, since movement attracts attention and alerts visually oriented predators such as birds. There are at least two ways caterpillars have evolved to reduce their risk of predation. Those prized as food by birds are highly camouflaged, and they hide and/or move very slowly, traveling to and from their feeding places only at night. They include the underwing or *Catocala* moth caterpillars, which feed in the crowns of trees at night and in the daytime hide on or in bark crevices on tree trunks and are practically invisible to us. Other fast movers, such as the arctiid woolly bear caterpillars, are spiny and bristly; most predators avoid them because they are presumably unpalatable, so they can safely be seen out and about in the open in the daytime.

The range of options evolved by insects gives us a view into the evolution and selective pressures of potentially vulnerable prey in the context of ever-present strong selective pressure by predators. Those predator-prey selective pressures have extended over a hugely longer time period for them than for mammals. Some insects stay in place and rely on camouflage. In sharp contrast, others more analogous to "protohominid" venture out into the open, running and capturing widely scattered food, a strategy seemingly copied from one of my childhood beetle favorites, the *Laufkäfer* (running beetles). Directly outside our tent in Botswana's Okavango Delta one evening, I saw one especially huge member of the genus *Anthia* running so fast that it appeared to be floating over the sandy ground. It is commonly called the "saber-toothed ground beetle," and aside from its sharp mandibles, it has a chemical weapon: the ability to spray a jet of formic acid up to 30 centimeters to blind potential attackers. It is black and fringed in shining white, clearly evolved to be noticeable, so it is seldom obliged to defend itself, because its defense capacity is well known. Our guide strongly advised me not to grab it, knowing perhaps that I had a strong temptation to do just that.

Caterpillars, beetles, some reptiles, birds, and mammals including us are born with these running speeds as a result of natural selection working mostly on body build, in the same way that greyhounds are fast and dachshunds slow. Iditarod dogs have great endurance compared to most other dogs, mainly due to their spirit and eagerness to run. Selection for running was not all based on VO_2 max, to which we attribute much of the variability in human running ability and that declines steeply with age and/or decline in physical exertion.

Aerobic training in insects is not something I had thought about, even when I was regularly measuring the oxygen consumption and/or metabolic rates of moths and bumblebees. As in birds, insects' energy cost in flight rises steeply when they are carrying a load, and it declines sharply when they are artificially made lightweight in flight (by suspending them so that they are no longer holding their own body weight aloft). One way they have evolved to minimize the otherwise heavy energy cost of transport by flight is by increasing their wing size, reducing their wing-beat frequency, and capitalizing on their sailing capacity. But even then, the minimum rate of contraction of their power-producing wing muscles (wing-beat frequency) is still much higher than that of our leg muscles, i.e., our maximum step frequency while running. A sphinx moth, for example, has a wing-beat frequency of fifty to a hundred times per second, while our running limb has a frequency of about four steps per second. We do not have the aerobic capacity to function at the high limb-frequency level. The question then is, how do insects do it? Is there something special physiologically in their muscles that we lack but might tap into? Even more astounding, why do we need extensive training to acquire our relatively puny capacity, whereas a moth or a bee, fresh out of its mummylike existence encased in a carapace and some in a cocoon, is virtually, in a wing beat, able to take off at full flight and contract its muscles to beat its wings at more than a hundred times a second? Don't their muscles, like ours, need training? I had always considered the question to be a theoretical one. How can one know?

It seemed obvious that a moth can't train its flight muscles to the exercise required an hour after emerging from its pupa and then its cocoon, and then live only several days. The pupa has no appendages and is packaged tightly into the cocoon of silk that the caterpillar spun around itself to protect itself from predators, and it may stay thus tightly wrapped for nearly a year until the time is right for it to crawl out, spread its soft inflatable wings, release a hormone from the brain that will result in hardening them, and then fly at or very near full capacity, in an hour or less.

Since I was about ten years old, I have hunted caterpillars to raise them to the adult stage, but I had never given their seemingly instantly superior aerobic performance a thought until the spring of 2020, while working on this book, when I happened to have a cocoon of a live luna moth pupa on the windowsill next to my desk, of a caterpillar that I had found the previous summer.

After the caterpillar had spun its silk cocoon during the late summer, I had left it outside in a wire screen cage through the fall and winter, along with other overwintering cocoons. Finally, in late April, I took it into my cabin, expecting that the warmer temperature would serve as a signal to override its circadian and/ or circannual clock and trigger its development and then elicit the emergence of the adult. I had not been paying any attention to it, because I didn't expect to see its huge pale green wings flutter until several hours after it had shed the hard exoskeleton of its pupa and then escaped from its cocoon. But on May 19, nearing the circannual time schedule of moth emergence, I heard a faint one- or two-second rustle from the cocoon, the twirling of the pupa's abdomen, the only part of it that can move, rubbing against the dry papery cocoon enclosing it. The next day I heard it again.

A fresh pupa contains what looks like liquid mush. But this one was obviously well on its way to containing an adult moth that might soon escape first from its pupal casing of chitin and then from its silken but solid-walled cocoon. Having just been thinking of animal exercise and longevity, the sounds alerted me to the possibility that the pupa might be exercising to get flight ready, and if so, there should be repetitive bouts of it in the days before the emergence when the moth would take flight, only to die soon after.

Now I started paying close attention, and the next day, there were fifteen episodes of the same scratchy one-to-two-second twirls; and I spent sixteen hours near the cocoon to record the clock time of every one of them. The next day, in fifteen hours, there were twenty-three episodes. Three days later, the moth, a male, emerged. However, due to his slightly accelerated development in temperatures that were higher than those outside, he was desynchronized from the biological times of any potential mates that he could have mated with. He had, however, an inordinate urge to fly, as if there were mates to be found, but he did that only at night when fluttering about, as dictated by his circadian clock. There were no leaves out yet and no females flying. But he lived out almost all of his natural adult life (of about three days) flying without any possible conscious knowledge of why, potentially responsive to a certain scent, one not encountered.

The moth's pupal exercise bouts and his then flying reminded me of us high school cross-country runners at an age when running felt most natural. We had no idea why or how we did it. We never gave it a thought; we just felt like doing it. There was no reason. Although Coach had guided our development, we were motivated by our own natural desires. Possible rewards or consequences would be indirect, unseen, and far into the future of a life to be lived.

14

The Hunt

WE TEND TO NOTICE THE TICKING OF THE BIOLOGICAL CLOCK by the effects it has in or on the body. But for us its impacts are also left on the mind. Their progression proceeds from one stage to another, leaving each behind as memories, and we are then often left in awe and wonder at what had been and how it had been possible. Now that I'm an elder, I've reached a new stage, one that earlier was unimaginable, as if of another world.

For me there was first the bug, butterfly, and beetle-collecting/hunting/acquiring phase, in which every form and species was a revelation that kicked up the brain's happiness chemicals, the endorphins. That stage never left entirely but morphed in my thirties into the hunt-for-scientific-discoveries stage, which provided thrills, perhaps because by then they could be and were shared with others to be appreciated by them also. Everyone could understand the excitement of an arduous journey through a wilderness of facts to reveal a marvel that did not exist before in human consciousness. The discovery might be the mechanism of a tiny moth regulating a higher body temperature than our own, by an anatomy entirely different from ours. It might be derived from simple observations that reveal some caterpillars that seemingly carelessly waste food but are instead discarding evidence of their presence, which reduced the odds of them being eaten by potential predators. For me it was a huge thrill to see how ravens share valuable food on the basis of self-serving actions, establishing definitive proof that they can think beyond the standard instinctive programmed responses and the expected learned ones, and are able to distinguish the three in controlled experiments. But long before making those discoveries, there is the intervening stage of beginning adulthood, marked by independence and a drive toward self-sufficiency that was at times expressed in what seemed like rebelling without rhyme or reason. It is, however, perhaps instead an expression of the driving force to be free, to explore, and to be somewhere new and different.

In the early stages of the biological clock that drives our lives, notions of wanting freedom may be expressed in the context of some excuse or rationalization. What is amazing in retrospect is how strong the desire can be and how flimsy and weak the logic required to act on it. The earlier the age, the less having a specific and suitable target is required. Indeed, we can invent targets from sheer imagination. And forget about consequences! Those didn't exist. They are the unknown future that leans not so much on facts but on wishes and rationalizations. As one prominent example of that discord, I'll never forget the first time Phil Potter took me deer hunting at the age of about fourteen years, shortly before I was sent to the Good Will School. We went into the woods at the foot of Bald Mountain, a mile from where I live now, planning to come out several miles to the west side of it by his and his wife, Myrtle's, tar paper–covered shack, their "camp." On our way through miles of beech, maple, and oak woodland, we encountered fresh deer hoofprints, and also the antler scrapes of rutting bucks; I could see the deer in my imagination and expected one to appear at any minute. And then, up ahead on the other side of some brush, I suddenly saw a buck standing still. I excitedly pointed it out to Phil: "There— there—by that big maple. See?" No, he could not see it. Finally, he handed me his .30–30 Winchester lever-action rifle, took it off safety, handed it to me, and said, "You shoot!" I saw the brown fur and the antlers, aimed, and pulled the trigger. *Bang!* "Get 'im?" he asked anxiously. No. Nothing had budged. "Shoot again!" Same result. Only then came the revelation, after we had moved closer: I had shot at dried fern and twigs, as my imagination had painted a deer out of them. The immature mind can invent a thing and then believe in it, if it wants it badly enough, and be wildly misguided. It can also believe appropriate lies, those in line with our wants and wishes, and strongly enough to cause damage. There can be no peace, or progress, without doubt to generate truth.

Three years later, the typically juvenile mismatch between wishes and facts happened to me again. This time the outcome was—thanks to sheer luck—wildly positive (for me) but caused by unanticipated random events. It concerned the same woods where I had been so enamored of the deer tracks and the fresh claw marks of bear on the nut-bearing beech trees that I wanted to live there. My vague plan, or more accurately a wild dream, was to make a log cabin in those woods, hunt deer and maybe a bear, and have a tame crow as a companion. Those thoughts seemed, in my mind then at seventeen, plausible, since I was then feeling a captive at the Good Will School and wanted out.

And so, with two other like-aged and like-minded buddies, I set off to live in those woods, leaving one night in early spring, with each of us carrying enough food to last at least a day or two. We had no thought about specifics beyond living in the woods. We traveled in the dark to avoid the state police, and two days later we did make it to the planned interim stop, our farm, where I planned to pick up my .22-caliber rifle while my mother was off to work in town (my father was then working in Ottawa). But although we made it that far, we were then apprehended because I was testing out my gun after we had had a nip of my mother's red wine. We considered ourselves clever and foresighted by replacing the reduced volume in the bottle with water. The result: my two friends were sent back to school, where we all belonged. I was declared the ringleader of the escapade and was kicked out, and so as "punishment" got to stay home on our farm. Having been kicked out for a year, I now attended the local public high school, Wilton Academy, as a sophomore. Best of all, my dream had come true. I had never been happier. I was free, lining bees, watching the woodcock dance in the sky over our fields, fishing, and knowing I would hunt deer in the fall.

In the woods of western (and southern, eastern, and northern) Maine, the "kudu" prey of the aspiring natives like myself is the white-tailed deer. Our method, however, is not running it down physically, as the San/Bushmen do, but hunting for it by sight, sound, and tracking on snow if present, day after day after day, in and through the endless woods, all the while carrying a high-powered rifle.

"Getting your deer" was then the unspoken and unwritten but well-understood rite of passage for a rural Maine teenage boy. An elder, usually the male parent, would take the boy to the favorite woods of his youth and show the aspiring one the fresh buck-antler scrapes on a sapling, the foot scrapes under a hanging fir bough, the hoofprints in a tangle of freshly fallen leaves, so all of them might ignite his hunting passion. Day after day after that intoxication the boy would go out, his mind aflame and alert to the electrifying sight of a white tail flag in the distance, the sound of the crack of a broken twig, or the subtle sign of a recent footprint.

Our neighbor Phil Potter, who paid me to do his farm chores a year or two after my shooting at an imagined deer, thought I had advanced to the next stage: going out alone. He instructed me that although the .22 I then owned was fine for the rabbits and "partridge" (ruffed grouse) I hunted, it would never do for a deer, and he again loaned me his .30–30 lever-action Winchester. And thus, during that fall of 1957, while I attended high school in Wilton, I was out hunting in the woods by our farm every morning before school and again after school. Again and again I would see signs but no deer. But then one morning it happened: suddenly up ahead, as I peered through the screen of a stand of tamarack trees, there stood a deer. My heart pounding, I raised the .30–30 to my shoulder.

I was so excited that all detailed memory is now blotted out, except that I went on autopilot, firing shot after shot. And then there lay the deer! I had to hurry off to school and get the word out. That was News. It felt like a life event, and I remember it as if it happened yesterday. I immediately had two volunteer helper classmates, Buddy York and Bruce Richards, who were eager to help me after class, and we went out together into the woods to retrieve my deer. We hung it from a pole and carried it out. It was a small one, as white-tailed deer go, but the point was the news: I had "got my deer." My mother took a picture of us carrying it into the barnyard, and it remains a treasured memory.

As I look back, I am impressed by how scanty the evidence had to be for me (or us in general) to act at that age. That hair-trigger response for perhaps large things with little deliberation comparing the pros and cons, that is to say irrationally, was and is dangerous. Stunts like that from the perspective of the present seem bizarre, though they felt perfectly natural then. I was therefore not surprised to encounter the precise phenomenon later in overeager researchers eyeing flimsy data with wide-open eyes, looking for what they wanted to see and then seeing it. I felt lucky to have hopefully learned from my own experience. No nonroutine behavior is without risk, but almost any change can under appropriate circumstances result in improvement and cannot be anticipated. It comes mostly by accident as one ranges far and wide. But the older I became, the more I leaned in the opposite direction, trying to stick to the proverbial tried and true, that which is possible. We rely on what we think we know, and therefore we can go no farther. And then it hit me why most of us have a specific age where we are most productive and creative, and also when we run and why.

Maturing mentally meant learning to make accurate judgments as to what is possible and what is not, and the huge implications of knowing the difference. I need more and more to know that the odds are in my favor before I invest. Going out hunting, I feel that the "deer" here now are more symbolic of "fat chance." I'm now in a different world from the idyllic pastoral one of chasing antelope because of being genetically imprinted to do so during our evolution on the African veldt, and also from the learning of long ago on the farm. I was a hunter once and young, but I'm older now and have for a long time not put much effort into deer hunting. Bringing home the venison hasn't meant much after the instincts damped down, and I can buy food at the grocery store at any time. Am I too old to be a passionate hunter as well as a runner? Perhaps the lessening of my previous burning passion is part of the general process of aging. Or is it still there and just needs to be reawakened by renewed contact? I thought I'd try to revisit the place, the season, and the activity of youth and try a deer hunt with my nephew, Charles H. Sewall (son of Charles F. Sewall, who was my handler in the twenty-four-hour run in Brunswick), in the only place where we ever hunt—the woods near our camp in Maine.

It is the last Saturday of November 2019, the last day of the Maine deer hunting season. Charlie was out the cabin door at dawn while I was still asleep. I get up late, brew coffee, and leisurely drink a cup, hang out about camp and do some scribbling while reclining on the couch, and then, instead of doing my usual four-mile morning run, decide to do a longer route, six miles, instead. Afterward I have another leisurely cup of coffee, and finally, near noon, I walk out, determined to spend an hour at "the rock."

This for us common destination is a house-sized, glacier-rounded precipice overshadowed by several mature hemlock trees at the edge of an open slope of never-logged hardwoods with an understory of hobblebush that is aglow with white flowers in spring but all bare of leaves now. It is a favorite spot that we hunt from, usually in rest, leaning against a thick hemlock tree after having spent the previous hours exploring from the swamps to the oak-and-spruce-clad ridges. I've been at the rock for a short session almost every day now for a month, staying for only an hour each time, collecting data on winter-flocking birds, and I plan to do the same today. It is a bucks-only season this year, and a snowstorm of four to six inches is forecast.

Tiny snowflakes are already starting to drift down as I walk the north trail to the rock, and by 1:00 p.m. a dusting covers the ground, enough to see tracks. I clamber up to our seat to sit out the hour, protected from the falling snow by the spreading hemlock. Week-old snow is still on the ground in the woods below, but it shows no tracks. Bummer, I think; there is not much to expect. But it is the last day of the hunting season, and I decide to stay the full hour.

The stillness is absolute. The only thing I hear and then see is a hairy woodpecker that keeps tapping here and there; no squirrels, no raven call; nothing is moving. Okay, I've done it. Another deer season is past, but with only five more minutes to wait, I stand up, and after a couple of minutes—was that a crack I just heard from upslope? Did a branch fall from the weight of the newly fallen snow? I'm about to sit back down when there is another distinct crash. It's definitely not a branch. I look upslope, and there, at full speed, comes a deer bounding downslope through the forest of beech, maple, and balsam fir. It's fast, and I have to look closely at the big ears sticking up to see if there might be a young buck's spike horns, too. I see none. It's a doe. But there is suddenly another crash, and right behind her comes a buck, one carrying a big antler rack.

He is now in the open, making huge leaps as I try to see him through the peep sights of my .30–30 lever-action rifle, the one Phil Potter gave me when I was seventeen because he'd purchased a new rifle with a telescopic sight and wanted to get rid of this old-fashioned piece belonging to a previous age. But this by now ancient rifle has become tradition, and it is still the only deer rifle I've ever used. I like it. A semiautomatic with telescopic sights would serve me better at the moment, as the deer is running fast and will be gone in three seconds. I fire off a shot, jack in another shell, shoot again. The buck is now over a rise and out of sight, heading downhill into a thicket of evergreen trees. I run over to check the track where he vanished: there is a drop of blood on the snow!

One might ask why a nature lover would want to kill a deer.

Isn't that an anachronism from our ancestors' lives as killer apes, cavemen, and/or mindless children? So I digress here at this point to ponder the issue, starting with one of the most profound nature quotes I know. It is from Henry Beston, who wrote these immortal words: "We need another and a wiser and perhaps a more mystical concept of animals. . . . They are not brethren, they are not underlings; they are other nations, caught with ourselves in the net of life and time, fellow prisoners of the splendour and the travail of the earth." Yes, they are other nations. That is why they are so fascinating. And no, I do not at this point in my life find myself more distant from them. Instead, I find myself closer. That is because I have seen my father sleeping with a bear cub, and my mother with her dearly loved monkey riding on her shoulder; have had crows, owls, wild geese, and ravens as companions, lived with a raccoon, a skunk, and several dogs. I have nurtured innumerable caterpillars to adulthood, and routinely fed chickadees from my hand. I am an advocate of close interspecies associations through mutual, not just one-way, interactions. Ingesting them is about as intimate as it gets, and I have eaten many mice, squirrels, and chickens, and would never pass up roadkill unless I had to. Eating other life is what every one of us does, every day. I don't think I would mind being eaten myself. I would, however, mind my death, knowing its finality. I would not mind so much if I were going into hibernation like a woodchuck, or frozen in a cube of ice in the fall only to be thawed out alive the next spring like a wood frog. I believe we are the only animal on the planet that can fear death. To all the others it is a secret; they cannot fear it. Dying is hard, but being eaten is no trial. In hunting, my main concern is to make the killing as painless as possible, and to eat every scrap of every animal killed. I believe we cause more suffering to any animal we eat if the bacon or chicken had all its life suffered in a cage. When killed in the wild, the animal suffers by our hand only once, hopefully for only seconds. A cardinal sin of hunting is to leave a wounded animal suffering.

The chase is on; a switch has been turned on in my brain as if I've just heard "On your mark, get set, go!" The only other deer my hunting partner Charlie and I have seen so far this fall was a dead one. It was on a patch of ground that was all torn up, with blood spattered onto the fallen leaves where we saw the head of a spike-horn buck poking out of a leaf pile. Coyotes or a bear had killed and eaten most of it and then covered up the rest.

After I follow the buck's track for ten minutes, I see him far ahead, taking fifteen- to twenty-foot bounds. He is not much hampered in his gait, but I have in years before seen one that after a heart shot, running hard dropped dead after a hundred yards, having run until oxygen depletion like a sprinter near the end of the 100-meter dash. This buck is going strong, running aerobically like a distance runner. But after sprinting and bounding downhill a couple hundred yards, he lay down briefly and left several more blood spots. He then jumped up and ran on, apparently because he sensed me on his trail.

A test of endurance is developing. Might I perhaps catch up to him? Or will he always be able to keep far enough ahead for me to never see him and get another shot? He leads me through woods I've never been in before: downhill into swamps, through thickets, then again to rock ledges, and down once more. I continue on the trail another hour, wondering if perhaps somewhere I have inadvertently crossed over from his track to another buck's, because there has been no shortening of his stride, and then I again find a single tiny red spot and know I'm still on his spoor.

And then the impossible: I'm hurrying along his trail at the

same time as I'm trying to look far ahead—the snow a clear
and ever-deepening sheet in all directions—and suddenly there,
after a patch where the track was unclear due to grass, there is
no track. It just stops! I'm so flabbergasted that I look up, even
knowing that the buck could not have climbed a tree. Obviously,
he has backtracked. He has returned on his own track to an
opening of grass and brush where he became hard to follow, and
I missed his backtrack when I went by in a hurry. Sure enough,
at that spot, his track led off at a ninety-degree angle but began
again only after a long leap. So now I follow that track, and
the same thing happens. Again I follow the trail, now heading
steeply uphill from old log cuttings and swamps into rugged
hills. I cross smoking hot fresh bear tracks where the leaves are
all scratched up under oak and beech trees, fresh turkey tracks
all around on the fresh snow as well. I'm receiving and unconsciously processing information in a steady stream, seeing and
feeling beyond what could be imagined and appreciating what is
revealed only by the doing and then the feeling.

The big buck has now led me to clamber up to near the top
ridge of Houghton Ledges, where Charlie shot his first buck
when he was a high school freshman at the same age as I was
when I shot my first, the fall I had hunted with Phil Potter.
Overlapping memories seem like rerunning the script, and now
I'm near the same place where Charlie and I raised our rifles and
both fired at once to get *our* deer. I am, as I was then, surprised by
all the activity inscribed on the snow there. The great gnarled old
red oak trees still stand, just as back then, due to their inacces-
sibility by logging vehicles. The oaks have again produced a good
mast crop, as they had on that memorable day forty years ago,
and the fallen leaves are all scuffed up by deer, bear, and wild
turkeys, which were absent from the Maine woods then. Now

with the new snow, the turkeys' search for acorns is all the more conspicuous. Nearly all the acorns will be eaten. There is competition for them among the deer, bear, turkeys, and squirrels. The coyotes will kill those that don't get enough, and weaken like I did in the Spartathlon.

The turkeys have been gathering the last of the fallen nuts, to make fat that will help them produce heat and survive the next five months of lean times in subfreezing temperatures. Surely our harvest of venison, an indirect bounty of the trees, links us to them in a bond to the land. We are excited by the animals that provide our livelihood, just as the deer, bear, and turkeys are by the acorns that are the gift of the land to us all. I'm not averse to eating deer instead of beef; the deer link me bodily and spiritually to the land.

The sky has meanwhile become ever more thickly clouded and dark, and it has been snowing ever more heavily and steadily, without a break. It suddenly occurs to me that I have not the faintest idea where I am. I've been practically running at a steady pace for at least two hours, and in only one more hour it will be pitch dark under a clouded sky. I stop and look around. I cannot see the sun, moon, or anything else from which to get a bearing. I have a disquieting thought: I might have to spend the night in the woods and of necessity I must leave the buck's track and try to get home. But where has the buck led me? In what direction might the cabin be and how far? A steep rise ahead of me seems familiar. But as I climb all the way up, I see that no, it is totally unfamiliar! I am lost. Night is approaching. There is only one possible solution: I have to backtrack.

Back down I rush, tracking myself, and it quickly becomes a race against the celestial clock, with the descending darkness and the falling snow. I think of many things, but mostly of getting home.

Surprisingly, I have so far felt no fatigue, despite my run in the morning, when I felt myself extending more than I wanted to. Here there is no question: I *have* to overextend myself. My body offers no resistance. It goes on and on, with no diminishing of pace.

Earlier this fall I climbed a nearby mountain with two friends. One was a veteran of that mountain and a Maine sports champion who showed his mettle by staying ahead of both of us, as this deer did of me, all the way up to the top of the mountain. But then, on the way down, he became weak and could not stand upright. We had to hold him up in order for him to put one foot in front of the other. It was merely his age. He was in his early seventies. And I'm almost eighty. In these steep hills, this is a race. Getting to the finish at the end of it is not just desirable; it is urgent. It has real value. It is not symbolic.

The snow keeps filling in the tracks left hours earlier, but I keep moving ahead before they fill entirely. I finally track myself back to "the Rock," where I started the chase, and then hit the north trail running south, back to the cabin in the dark. I run it all the way.

That was "trail running" on the deer's trail, but it was mostly off trail in snow, on steep slopes, wearing boots, carrying a rifle, and it had been a blast. It was, I now realized, also an unanticipated experiment in the physiology of endurance. I wondered if I could have caught up with the buck that had outrun me if I had been younger and faster. I'm long past my peak. And had my life depended on the outcome, with natural selection at work, I would have lost and the buck would have won. But as it was, I did win by not collapsing; I made it home safe and sound to be able to run another day. I had unconsciously paced myself to run the way that felt right, not to achieve a specific clock time, and had therefore adapted my body to parcel out energy to sustain a rate that allowed it to stay the course.

I had in the last month slacked off in my running, doing no more than about 30 miles per week. My daily body (sublingual) temperature had remained mostly near the slightly subnormal (but normal for me) 97.7 to 97.8 degrees F range (as opposed to the official norm of 98.6 to 98.8 degrees). The evening after the deer chase it was 97, in my normal range. But the sublingual temperature did not tell the whole story; the peripheral temperatures revealed more. At 7:10 p.m., in the warm cabin (72 degrees), my hands and feet, even in long underwear and socks, felt cold. Though my mouth temperature was 97.5 degrees, the temperature in the crook of my arm was 95.2 degrees and that in the crook of my bent knee was 94.8 degrees. When I held the tip of the thermometer between my fingers or inserted it between my toes, the fancy thermometer, which beeps when it has made a reading, did not beep at all; the temperature was too low for it even to recognize.

I had for many years been routinely taking my sublingual body temperature, along with my heart rate, sometimes many times per day and under all sorts of circumstances, to compare them with my observations of insects. I was, as before, using myself as a guinea pig to probe the relationships among body temperature, energy expenditure, and energy balance in the comparative biology of animals in general. Like my low resting heart rate in the mid to high thirties per minute, my normal body temperature at rest is also low and approaches the listed "normal" only after I eat a large meal, reminiscent of a mild version shown normally by large cold-blooded reptiles; their body temperature is low and also increases after they ingest a large meal. Similarly, I had in one of my studies of bumblebees found a huge decline in their muscle temperatures when they were foraging from flowers providing only small amounts of sugar in their nectar. That greatly reduced their foraging speed and extended the time of their foraging trips. Perhaps my body had also been trained to conserve calories in response to having had small reserves since early childhood. I still vividly recall the spot in the road in the forest where on my way walking or running back from school an epiphany hit me: the religious promised Paradise had to be where you could eat all the fried chicken you wanted to. I had at that time recently tasted chicken since Papa had caught one and came back to our Hahnheide hut with it. He said it had been running wild in the woods, and the taste of it when Mamusha had cooked it had been a rare and memorable pleasure.

I recall an old scientific paper comparing the thermal responses of the Atacama Indians of Patagonia, who, unlike the scientists studying them, slept nearly naked on the ground and seemed comfortable despite having very low foot temperatures. The authors concluded that the Indians had evolved this way as an adaptive strategy for energy conservation. However, it is also plausible that it was a learned brain mechanism for conserving energy. Not allocating calories to heat production may save them to burn in the future, such as for hibernation or finishing a long race.

In chasing the deer, I had done nearly what our Paleolithic ancestors had done for millions of years. They had not tried to outrun just any prey at any time. They incapacitated it or hunted during the heat of the day, when they had the thermal advantage.

They of course used weapons, including poison, with which they could wound the prey to slow it and then pursue it for a shorter distance before it had to stop. The possibility of my not catching up to the deer by night and then not surviving the night was not remote. Natural selection has for us likely been working to enhance endurance physiology by sparing energy as opposed to blasting it out for pure speed.

Speed can be increased with practice under optimal conditions and with ample food. But in the long run, food depletion and prolonged energy expenditure are countered by dampening down the growth rate (along with a likely associated slower aging rate later). I was within half a year of being eighty years "old" and I was not yet over the hill, but that buck turned out to be more of a challenge than I had imagined. I now planned to eat more when I feel like it to keep up my body temperature and speed, at the same time doing an occasional mock deer chase, maybe even running an official trail race.

15

On a Nature Trail

AT AGE EIGHTEEN, RUNNING FELT MOST VISCERAL AND PRI-
mal in all its power, simplicity, and purity. As we grow older, we
act for purpose rather than for pleasure, geared perhaps toward
achieving a reward or trinket like lab rats pushing a lever for a
food pellet. Pandering to that model, running in races used to be
cheapened by fake-gold so-called trophies that take up space on
a shelf, when the real rewards are the pleasures and treasures in
the mind. However, it was and is perfectly okay that watching
an ultramarathon is as exciting as watching paint dry, because we
runners do not need to spill our guts to please anyone. Running
is contact with the real and, because it demands effort, is often
associated with acute discomfort. Nevertheless, the contentment
of rest cannot be felt without a backdrop of experienced exhaustion. Pleasure in running is reminiscent to me of the pleasure of
sidling up to the fire in a stove after experiencing the routine of
a long, cold winter day.

I had not felt true contentment, such as after running an
ultramarathon, for a long time but had over several years raced
in two 10k's every fall. For training I had daily run a four-mile
route, out the cabin door and down a rocky path, a mile along a
tarred road, and then off onto a sandy side road to a bridge over

a brook and back. An ultramarathon was far from my mind. Been there, done that. That is, until Jason Mazurowski, a student, friend, and ultramarathoner, casually told me about one.

He described the race to me as "on mostly rolling hills on rural back roads." I envisioned farmhouses, fields of goldenrod and yellowing grass, forests of reddening maples in a bucolic Vermont countryside of meadows and cow pastures, reviving also the nostalgic image of my very first ultramarathon, the 50k held in nearly the same location forty years earlier that had ignited the ultramarathon fire in me. It seemed fateful if I were to be back, to complete the circle and run my last ultramarathon at nearly the same time, distance, and place. And so it was that I stepped up to the starting line of the Brownsville 50k at 8:00 a.m. on Sunday, September 29, 2019, the tag identifying me as number 1486 pinned onto my shirt. That was by far the largest number I had ever worn, and I realized that this could be unlike any ultramarathon I had ever run.

There were 243 registered runners, of whom 111 were women. In my previous races there had been perhaps thirty to forty participants, and they had almost always been mostly men. This time there was no command of "On your mark, get set, *go!*" for the start, so it was not important for me to be in the front row to take advantage of every second recorded by the timer's stopwatch at the end. This race was advertised as one "to enjoy a challenging and scenic Vermont landscape course." What? Race to enjoy the scenery? What *is* this?

In less than a mile we were laboring up a steep hill along a narrow dirt path with steep drop-offs to one side and winding in tight loops and switchbacks; it was the roughest trail I could imagine, even for hiking. As we wound through the woods, over bare roots and among loose rocks and boulders, there were

45-degree uphills and downhills. We had to watch every step. The switchbacks were so tight that at one point a runner behind me called me back because he thought I was heading in the wrong direction. So I went back, but it then turned out I had been right the first time and had done the same distance twice. The same course was simultaneously occupied by a separate fifty-mile trail race, plus a third race, a fifty-mile bicycle race. Sharing the path with bicycles racing down upon you from above and behind required stepping off to avoid collisions. As the cyclists came careening downslope they were hollering "Left!" or "Right!" to indicate which way you should move but without saying whether they were coming by *at* that side or you should step *to* that side. Perhaps there had been instructions, which I had of course not read. Clearly, finishing time was irrelevant. This was no race against the clock, and I gladly stepped off the trail entirely every time, to let them all pass. Invariably each rider said "Thank you" or "Much appreciated," something I had never before heard in a race.

As the runners and bikers careened on, I more crawled than ran up and down along the mountainsides, down the steep winding slopes and over stone walls of abandoned farms. It was unlike anything I had ever done or even imagined. It was more like my slightly later, barely possible deer hunt, but this one with assured beer instead of a deer promised at the end.

Unlike in any deer chase, there were pleasant and welcome compensations, as local people had provided aid stations along the way. A party atmosphere prevailed, and all sorts of food and drink were offered, including pickle juice—a new one to me. Eventually I heard loud music as I approached one station that from a distance I thought meant the finish-line festivities. But once there, I was informed that there were "only fourteen more miles." I was already near exhaustion and stumbled on at an ever-slower pace, trying to stay upright and not stub my toe on a root to be flipped downslope against the rocks. The course would have made excellent hiking trails except that hiking trails go from one destination to another. This one did not. It would end where it had started. But what we were encountering was no secret. Had I read the course description before coming, I would have stayed home. It read "Alpine slopes" and "If you get lost you must go back on your own to the spot you went off course" (did that), and "Total vertical of 5,600 feet," along with "A climb of a 1,600 feet attention getter" (no kidding) and "Fairly decent footing" (for mountain goats?) but "Rocks and roots," "Base to peak mountain climb," and "Gnarly peak to peak challenge." All of that.

A revolution had happened since my old running days. The goal of this extravaganza was different from any I had known. It was no longer to achieve a win or a good time for the distance. Neither time nor distance were relevant. Here, distance was a deliberate impediment, just like all the rocks, roots, loops, precipitous slopes, and sometimes weather. Only the last was excluded here. This day the weather was perfect, but that was by accident.

The point was to make not one thing but practically everything difficult. The goal here was to triumph over adversity, and finishing was no mean achievement, as proven by the forty-four participants who dropped out despite the perfect weather. The difficulties were by design. *They* make the achievement, for without them there is no such thing as accomplishment. Meanwhile, everyone was supposedly "having fun" or trying to convince themselves they were—maybe taking in the scenery?

I was experiencing something from a new era, my first trail

run. I had to walk at times, as did others. But stopping to walk here was not considered quitting. It was not shameful. Again and again in the latter part of the race while I ran stumbling and bumbling along, I was passed, and the passers one after another said, "Nice going!" or "Good job!" No, no, no, I was barely surviving. My only goal, after a while, was indeed just to finish.

Finally, when I could see the foot of the mountain where I thought the finish *might* be and it seemed I might even make it—*if* I really tried hard. But it turned out that it was a (deliberate?) illusion; there was still another three-mile loop to go that once more led first up and then down the mountainside, and then back to the afore-presumed finish, one that loomed ever larger as a sort of Shangri-La. What an incomparable relief to finally see it up ahead and to somehow still be able to run the last hundred yards.

After that race, due to stiffness and aching pain in both knees, I could not walk for hours and was left with one thought: don't do this again. Nevertheless, there was also the huge satisfaction in having done it. Simply having finished canceled out the pain of exhaustion in minutes, and to my surprise and joy, my knees were perfectly fine the next day.

Ultrarunning is a young person's sport, and now it is also as much a woman's as a man's game. The first woman, Lucy Skinner, age twenty-six, finished second overall, beating all but one man. As would be expected, of the first thirteen finishers, all but one were in their twenties and thirties, reminding me of my boyhood hero, the unbeatable Aussie Herb Elliott, who quit running at age twenty-two. My official time was accurate to a hundredth of a second, but it was as irrelevant to me as for everyone else. Due to the variability between trail courses, any "record" in a trail race can refer only to that specific course. Of the 182 runners who finished, I finished 143rd, having outrun 16 percent of those aged twenty to forty-nine years of age and 30 percent of those fifty to sixty-nine years, but I placed first of anyone seventy years old or over—in fact, I was the oldest person to finish the race by a margin of ten years. I could still run with the crowd and was thankful for it.

More than a race, the event was a worship ceremony. It was fittingly held all day on a Sunday, reminding me of the Good Will School in Maine, where in my teens, after the required Sunday attendance in the chapel, I would run back to my residence, Pike Cottage, change out of my church uniform of neatly ironed white shirt, tie, and suit jacket into shorts and a T-shirt, then run out into the woods on nature trails to hear the music of the birds and see the beauty all around. Here in Vermont that Sunday the "church" building was a big tent. There was no choir but instead a band. There was no preacher in a pew in a black robe giving a sermon but organizers wishing us all "a great run" and to "enjoy the natural beauty on this magnificent day." It was a meeting of minds and body, with live music and afterward a barbecue meal with complimentary beers.

I had experienced my first trail run, a new model of running, the sequel to running that used to be for state, national, and international titles, if not also records. Running long distance has morphed into a new experience, a model that combines the supporting of charities (through sponsorship funded by race entry fees), Nature appreciation (by being geared to the natural setting), health for everyone (everyone can choose his or her own goal), integration, and tolerance (as it is of course open and inviting to everyone regardless of age, gender, nationality, race, or belief). It either substitutes for religion or is becoming one, since it supports and promotes harmony and kinship with Nature, doing good, sympathy and concern for others as individuals, and a humbling to us as humans. We are part of a symbiosis with all of life, and the creatures we encountered were as well, and they were not insignificant in this new setting.

Ravens, using their specially designed front pair of limbs rather than our specially designed hind pair, had been flying overhead, swooping down the mountainside, catching the air, and winging their way up to do it again and again in the company of others of their kind, shouting at and with each other all the way in raucous voices we could never mimic, although they can and do mimic us. Blackpoll warblers (*Dendroica striata*), which live on mountains all over the North American continent, were just then gathering and starting to travel their own challenging traditional route, a three-day, 1,500-mile, nonstop, fly-or-die flight down the eastern seaboard and across the Gulf of Mexico to South America. Many of them would have already traveled across the continent from northern Alaska to the East Coast, never having done it before. In the spring they will take a different route, with a stopover in Florida on the way back to Alaska or to their spruce-topped home on a mountaintop in northern New England. They do it, we say, because they are migrating to escape winter, and in the reverse direction to come back to nest in the spring. But let us never forget: the ravens and the warblers do it for the same reasons we do, like us runners on the mountain that day: they do it because they feel like doing it. Period. And how did evolution make them feel like doing it? By linking the activity to a flow of endorphins that make it fun and, if important enough, irresistible. So it is for the joy of it, with no thought of an ultimate reward. They (at least the young of the year) cannot consciously know where, how, or why they are going because they have no language to transmit that knowledge to the adults. The ravens *feel like* plunging down like an arrow through the air, the warblers *feel like* flying with the wind at their tail rather than into it, and so they wait for that as the signal to start, just as we take off on our runs when we wait for and then hear "Go!"

16

Running the Clock

WHEN YOU ARE WITHIN THREE MONTHS OF THE AGE OF EIGHTY, there can still be running, but there is no longer *racing*, at least not with forty-year-olds. The biological clock does not allow it; it is instead your opponent. It enforces reasonable expectations of the finishing times one might aim for, which can be visualized on a graph, where you wonder if you can beat the numbers. Or more successfully you run for the sheer joy of running.

A graph in front of me from *UltraRunning*, in "The Aging Slowdown" by Peter Riegel, plots pace in minutes per mile of individuals' finishing times in fifty-mile races as a function of age. It gives a clear picture of what the clock does to you when it comes to running a fifty-mile distance.

The first thing you notice is, as expected, the stunning effect of age: from ten to eighty years of age there is a U-shaped pace curve from slow to fast and then back down to slow. The very best recorded finishing time of the youngest finishers at age ten is a nine-minutes-per-mile pace, and the last at age eighty is twelve minutes per mile. In between the curve dips to the world-record best at any age to just under five minutes per mile, which is at the age of twenty-eight years. The curve is smooth, and the bottom (fastest age-related) times over the full age range, in order of youngest to oldest, bear the names of Breinan (age 10), Cortez (age 15), Cortez (age 20), Klecker (age 28), Kirik (age 34), Heinrich (age 41), Corbitt (age 50), Ratelle (age 58), Casady (age 67), and Mostow (age 78). It seems significant that nowhere (except Cortez at ages 15 and 20) does the same name repeat in successive age ranges. The best for a nearby age beyond twenty is almost always a different person. That is, it looks as though one can reach the record chart either early or late in one short period of a lifetime—but it will not be as fast as that of someone who does *not* run records early, but who attempts his or her age-group record at a later age. Undoubtedly the names and the record times will change, but likely only a matter of seconds, and they will not affect the shape of the graph. There is for men, from ages thirty to fifty in the elite category, a decline of two to three minutes per year of the record times at the fifty-mile distance. After that the slowdown happens faster. And it is not just a slowdown: a subsequent article in *Ultrarunning*, "When Do Ultrarunners Stop Running Ultras?" by Pat McKenzie, shows that after age fifty-four, there are very few ultrarunners finishing at all, for both men and women. "For probably a variety of reasons" McKenzie concludes, "we stop running ultras," yet hedges with: "maybe because we are smarter." But, judging for myself, I tend to doubt the latter!

I ran my world masters record fifty-mile at age forty-one at an average pace of 6:38 per mile, while Ted Corbitt's record at age fifty-four was 7:52 per mile. Had he run that at age forty-one, he would or could have run it as fast as I did, and if I had raced instead at age fifty-four, I could have run close to his time, all else being equal. However, since record times are achieved only when everything is going just right, that makes them all close to being equal except for the age variable; if there had been a flaw or a weakness, there would have been no record. I ran another fifty-mile race for time at age sixty, nineteen years after my first US record. It was also a US age-group record, and my pace of 8 minutes per mile was 82 seconds per mile slower than at age forty-one, almost exactly on the same age-specific curve. According to the same graph, I should now at age eighty be able to run the fifty-mile (when I'm fully in shape and everything is going perfectly) at a pace of 14:30 per mile and thus should finish in about 12 hours and 15 minutes. However, that record is held by Bill Dodson of California, who ran much faster—a 10:16-per-mile pace—and who at age eighty holds all four of the major records, all of which he set in 2015 and 2016. I've been running over a spread of around sixty years and have spent it all, he for only half as many years; he didn't start racing until he was fifty years old. He had saved it for later, and thus to me his time seems physically as well as mentally beyond my reach.

Where have all the flowers gone, indeed? I was wondering that and trying to orient myself toward that question during my four-mile run earlier today, May 10, 2020. Long ago, I had many magical and unbelievable runs. They seem all the more wonderful precisely because they are not reachable now.

The past is gone, but each day's new opportunities are almost always built on the past. In his novel *And Quiet Flows the Don*, Mikhail Sholokhov took from the Cossack folk song "Koloda-Duda" the words "Where are the flowers? The girls have taken them. Where are the girls? They have taken husbands. Where are the men? They're in the army." Pete Seeger, while on a plane ride to visit Oberlin College, faintly remembered having read that earlier and made a song of it that was made famous by Joan Baez in the late 1960s: "Where have all the flowers gone, long time passing."

A long time has passed since the flowers of my racing days. Time has moved on. The flowers may have been picked or died, but their seeds can and hopefully are sprouting. That's what the clock does—for every living thing.

The biological clock causes trees to grow for a long time before they produce flowers and seed when they are old, as opposed to a daisy, which produces them in a year. The evidence of comparative biology shows longevity to be positively correlated with seeking to achieve reproductive capacity. In humans, reproduction is social, and the family unit may include grandparents, who throughout our history have helped to release their children to have more children. This helps promote the interests and lives of those we feel close to, a process powered by emotions generated in the brain that then affect our endocrine system. It's how we and other animals physically connect to our environment. But our emotions are also generated by thought aside from mere sensing.

A hundred feet from the log cabin I'm in, which is next to the one that I'd built with Maggie forty years earlier, a song burst forth that I had heard here only once, years before. As I lay in bed ruminating about what the clock was saying, I heard the resounding trisyllable "whip-poor-will" repeated over and over. It was 8:40 p.m., and it lasted almost two minutes. The rest of the night may have been silent, but at dawn, the pair of phoebes was again tending to their nest, decorating it with fresh green moss at its rim before laying their four or five pure white eggs. The birds' circannual as well as circadian clocks had activated their behaviors, setting into motion their migration, singing, mating, nest building, egg laying, incubation, and provisioning of young, each at its appropriate time, cued by environmental stimuli perceived by the senses and processed by the brain. The same will apply in the fall, when they leave to fly southward.

In his book *In Suspect Terrain*, John McPhee begins with a geological consideration of time in which time starts a billion years ago as a continent breaks apart to create an ocean where the Atlantic is now. In more recent times, at least a dozen ice ages have come and gone, and fifty more are expected to revisit perhaps all of Canada, New England, New York, Pennsylvania, and the Midwest. We are presently in a relatively deglaciated interval in which a still-to-come glacier two miles thick will, as McPhee writes, "pluck up Toronto and deposit it in Tennessee."

There is much time left. But only that which we can grasp can have relevance for us. Would we plant trees if we didn't think we were part of Nature and therefore promoting our own longevity? As Gina Rae LaCerva notes in *Feasting Wild*, "Every action is an ecological act." Our acts as adults are for most of us derived from thoughts rooted in physical reality. We have thoughts that other animals who rely mainly on emotions can't have. We therefore have possibilities of internally generated longevity, of selves that can extend not only to our roles in society but also into Nature, where we came from in deep time, as well as proximally after our personal longevity has expired.

17

The Church of Nature

THERE IS A ROUGH PINE-BOARD TABLETOP IN MY LOG CABIN, which Maggie and I built by hand in the summer I trained there for my 100k record. It is held up by two black cherry tree trunks with their bark on. Students of my winter ecology field course have sat at this table to eat our meals, to collate notes taken in the woods, and to discuss the fauna and flora. Afterward we often listened to the banjo and the fiddle by our multitalented members, as we joined in song and jumped up and danced wildly on the wooden floor in the light from a lamp and the warmth from the woodstove. We had scoured the woods daily, looking for birds, identifying trees, tracking mammals in the snow to try to get to know them. At some time in our annual twenty-four seven stay there, when we gathered in the evenings on two log benches on opposite sides of the table, we (and sometimes guests) carved their names, line figures, and perhaps a thought into the table's rough wooden top. One inscription from a former student carved on the southeast corner of this table reads: "Nature is God. The key to life is contact. Evolution is mother and father of mankind. Without them we'd be nothing."

All of us are derived from an ancient anomaly, a single cell-like structure. Then as now it most likely had DNA in which three uracil molecules in a row coded phenylalanine into protein chains. This was and is only a minuscule part of the magic of how it could copy itself and, once it did, repeat doing so indefinitely. That started more than 3.5 billion years ago and is still happening now, with anomalies and selective reproduction occurring in a process we now define as evolution.

Humans, Nature, society, and religious faith are strongly intertwined, and we have traditionally thought of ourselves as the crown jewel of creation, superior beings compared to the blue whale, the scarlet macaw, the ruby-throated hummingbird, the white-lined sphinx moth. We have only recently, in the last second of geological time, differentiated into our socio-technological niche from our apelike scavenging-hunting progenitors, whereas some of what we may consider the lowest animals, such as termites, have evolved their sociality from cockroaches millions of years before us. One might suppose termites provide lessons in what makes a social system work, inasmuch as ours at times seems imperfect. At least that was what the Harvard entomologist William Morton Wheeler (1865–1937) implied in his book *Social Life Among the Insects* (1923), where he states, "History shows that throughout the centuries, from Aristotle and Pliny to the present day, natural history constitutes the perennial rootstock or stolon of biological science and that it retains this character because it satisfies some of our most fundamental and vital interests in organisms as living individuals more or less like ourselves."

In an earlier whimsical, tongue-in-cheek 1920 essay in *Scientific Monthly* titled "The Termitodoxa, or Biology and Society," Wheeler had already broached the theme by inventing a hypothetical termite king named Wee-Wee, of the 8429th Dynasty of the Bellicose Termites (a real and common African species,

Termes bellicosus) colony. He posited that Wee-Wee should be given credit for being social at a much more pronounced level than we are, and endowed him with proficiency in the English language to instruct us in the ways termites have solved many of the same problems we face. These problems are generally recognized as those of nutrition, energy management, the environment, resources, enemies, military science, hygiene, child rearing, elder care, and longevity. Wee-Wee in his implied wisdom suggested that such problems *could* be solved in the human world, if we understood what termites do. But he posited that "would require us to increase our biological investigators a hundred fold, put them in positions of trust and responsibility," and pay them "at least as well as we pay plumbers and bricklayers" so that we can "look forward to making as much social progress in the next three centuries" as we have made "since the Pleistocene." He concluded with "the sincere wish" that some such opinion might also be entertained by some of our statesmen "sometime before the end of the present geological age."

The one thing both Wheeler and Wee-Wee left out is what termites have and we lack, which is that termite and other insect societies are held together as units by their common *scent*. Unlike a specific scent directing us, thought and imagination allow for the possibility of lies and make things much more variable and less cohesive. We do not have the convenience of one specific scent as a social unit identity, and we compensate mostly by complex behavior to identify and hence differentiate ourselves. Language is the main one, although color, clothing, hairstyles, and unique customs and/or religion can all contribute as well. Identification works well, except for the Faustian bargain that what unites also separates—the identity that distinguishes and unites us also creates "others," those who are evolutionarily and often traditionally perceived as competitors. They are those on the other side of the mountain or body of water whom we have to distinguish from our own group, in order to fight them better. That antipathy can be adaptive, as our love is strengthened and reserved for those of our group and our hate for the other; we fight best when we hate the most. Indeed, the more the others are a threat, the more we love those in our own group and vice versa. This creates evolution in a way in which *both lose*, as it accentuates differences and is difficult to extricate ourselves from, unless we are conscious and deliberately forgiving enough to counter the natural trend. How? As inscribed on that corner of the rough-hewn tabletop in my log cabin: "Nature is God. The key to life is contact." If Nature is wholeness, then it is effectively what all faiths aspire to be in tune with. The problem is the contact with it, in a mutual ceremony where all can participate, and I posit that running together, such as I experienced in my trail run, is a good place to start. It joins us all in something universal, fair, and ecologically as well as individually beneficial.

We are now recognizing more and more what we have in common. The tall mountains and the seas no longer separate us. We are rapidly converging on a global language, and, with new technology, we are able to communicate almost instantly across all barriers and distances. I will never forget one time standing with Erica, my daughter, along a remote stream in the Okavango Delta in Botswana. She pulled a thin little gadget out of her pocket and in seconds was talking with Gaberial and Liam, my grandsons, who were at that moment sitting in the kitchen of their home in Cape Elizabeth, Maine. There was no more "us" versus "them." Our safari leader could not be seen as different from a next-door neighbor from any city in the world just because he is an African. Before, we united for safety, to be better able to fight "them." Now "they," regardless of color, distance, or artificial political boundary lines, are a second away by a click of the internet all over the planet. We are becoming part of a single ever-converging swarm on an ever-shrinking lot, and our social nature dictates that we unite in Nature; it feels good to belong to and be a part of Nature, something much greater than ourselves, in a communal struggle against a perceived or real enemy. The common enemies that blot out or reduce our possible differences and unite us include poverty, environmental degradation, over-population, pollution, a virus, the decline and even extinction of species, global warming, and the inequitability and responsibil-ity of wealth, health, educational opportunity, and taxes. We are recognizing that we are all in the same lifeboat on and in the sea of Nature, having the same needs in a finite world of grand beauty governed by common constraints *and* possibilities.

We now recognize that there is a common enemy and that connecting with others is vital for us. We belong by belonging. Running the same races, singing the same songs, and having the same clothes and hairstyles may suffice. But running together on a trail in the mountains creates a special breed that is automati-cally united by the same goal—finishing a difficult course that winds in and through spectacular and beautiful Nature, with the challenges thereof added to bind the participants through that particular experience and with Nature and our roots in it.

Participating in a run creates a like-minded social group. Each knows the steep entry fee to the club. All know that they already have or will now pay their dues. And the greater the effort required, the greater the reward, and the more bonding takes place. All along the way, we cheer one another along as we fight to ascend and descend steep hills, hearing perhaps a raven calling overhead here, a red squirrel chattering there, but soon enough in our pain and agony, waiting to cross the finish line into the promise of a heaven of reward and satisfaction. Others' gain is not at our cost but rather a shared pleasure.

As befits our social nature, we unite in rituals, preferably in special places. These places become part of the rituals, and a great effort is made to maintain them as grand, beautiful, long lasting, and readily available. In the Middle Ages, such places were man-made cathedrals, still standing as symbols of the faith for many of the great religions. Wherever a religion goes, the places to worship go with it. Why not instead cultivate and use and worship in the sacred groves themselves, those made by Nature? John Muir worshipped in them, as did Henry David Thoreau and millions of others then and now; all those who get close enough to Nature feel its beauty, power, and majesty. However, we are highly social, and for us there was and perhaps still is one thing missing before Nature can be worshipped, and that is the human ritual of communal participation. For that I cannot think of anything better than running; it feeds the soul and the body, the seat of the soul.

Running has a set of values, is based on beliefs of excellence, and has rules for how we should behave. It has now become global; its rituals and beliefs unite us. In 1897, the Boston Marathon had fifteen finishers; in 2015, there was a more than two thousand–fold increase to 30,231. Participation in the New York City Marathon grew from 55 finishers in 1970 to 51,000 in 2016. The spectators at the Boston Marathon are estimated to now be near a half million. In the 1970s, there was seldom a runner on the street. Now they are part of the scene. Running clubs are springing up all over. In New York City, Kovon Flowers is the captain of Black Men Run, an organization with the goal of building a stronger community. The club was cofounded in Atlanta in 2013 by Jason Russell and Edward Walton to fight heart disease and stroke, the top killers of black men. At the time of writing it has fifty-three chapters nationwide. Its motto is "A Healthy Brotherhood." The process of getting into shape is moving from the gym to outdoor activities, to inculcate a fitness culture by providing opportunities for it.

Events celebrating the virtues of running are open to anyone. It is the one outdoor sport open and accessible to all regardless of economic means, race, gender, political affiliation, or any other orientation. It is available to the most deprived economically, because the biggest step is always the first out the door and onto a path, any path. There is no arena, no court, no club required, not even a pair of shoes. People have set records barefoot. It does not matter where participants live. Where there is a will, there is a way. Not only are all welcome, all can show up on equal footing to get onto the road to better health, including more neurons being produced by the brain, muscles being strengthened for more speed and endurance, and a potentially longer life span. There is joy at others' success. That makes it social, and one can tear up appreciating what it took for a great performance such as running the four-minute mile or the two-hour marathon, a young girl finishing a race, or a great run by an eighty-year-old grandmother. It is the beauty of excellence, seeing what can be done. That is what inspiration is, a source of the real that one can empathize with and join in spirit if not in body. We become one. That alone makes running precious, and all over the world, with the crowning events such as the Olympics every four years, it brings us all together as contestants in a glorious, global, nearly instant participation by proxy.

Religion is the result of the human need, derived from our social natures, to belong to something greater and beyond us that inspires awe and respect. It is a feeling based on our understanding of the world and our recognition of its beauty and splendor, our belief that it does not merely exist but has been made and thus we have been made part of it, as are the elephant and the meadow mouse. There is, then, in our understanding, an order to it all, an appreciation of where we fit in.

We live in an extraordinary time. At the end of the last century, there was an explosion of knowledge about life and the universe, knowledge that is now becoming universal. Charles Darwin had already fathomed this at age twenty-eight (long before his enlightenment about our origins) when he wrote, "If we choose to let conjecture run wild then animals our fellow brethren in pain, disease death & suffering & famine; our slaves in the most laborious work, our companion in our amusements, they may partake, from our origin in one common ancestor we may be all netted together." This concept of being netted together, promoting awe and respect, and guiding our behavior is the common underpinning of all religions faiths that had relied on myths and are strengthened by our recent profound insights on our natural world. One concept that evidence does not support is that the earth and all that is in it has been created for specifically our use and our benefit, at the cost of all others'. What we hold in appreciation and awe is that which we cherish, promote, and respect. We are now on that path. We are, whether we define it yet as such or not, beginning a new era, one of Nature faiths based on revealed facts. We are One with all of life as a fact. Our genetic unity with all of life makes us a part of a continuity, and as Edward O. Wilson explains in *The Future of Life* in reference to his biophilia hypothesis, "To conserve biological diversity for ourselves is an investment in immortality." Running with the "antelopes" figuratively, if not also literally, is the ritual of this assembly, in the church of Nature. Running is a ritual. As in a faith, it involves listening to and disciplining ourselves and each other. We perceive limits. We see bounds and we see ways.

Running in Nature is getting close to it, absorbing its magic. Proximity creates unity, tolerance, and respect, all achieved through personal satisfaction. There is reference to the Real. Call it Mother Nature or call it God. We are not born to subdue her or it. We are here to nurture her, for she made us and we return to her. We each continue in the life that really *is* everlasting. We are singular on this earth, but so are the wild boar, the bear, the tiger, and the monarch butterfly. There is no rational protocol by any authority to elevate one above the rest. We are equal in the calculus of Nature, but still act as though Earth were made just for us, as I was made visually aware during a flight at great height, seeing an unending expanse of crop circles below me where there had recently been prairies alive with millions of bison, wolves, antelope, birds, and insects, all living off an almost unimaginably beautiful and plentiful diverse life of plants. Gone.

Nancy Bowker, a Quaker contemplative, told me that she had been working in that area as a laborer, in a pumpkin patch where she "heard" from behind her: "If you listen to us it will be like freeing the slaves." She knew it was the plants speaking to her. A vocal pronouncement from plants, as she described it to me, sounds absurd because plants don't speak. But through science and ecology they do speak to us, figuratively and loudly, by the soil and what grows in it; by the weather that affects whole ecosystems, including oceans; and by the vast prairies converted to crop monocultures fed by toxic chemicals to grow our food.

Afterword

AS I LOOK BACK ONCE MORE TO EXAMINE THE ROUGH PINE-board tabletop in my log cabin, which Maggie and I built by hand in the summer that I trained for my 100k record, I glance at the now hundreds of initials, images, and dates carved there, and as always seem to return to the inscription that is now faded with time, yet the words remain clear and legible: "Nature is God. The key to life is contact. Evolution is mother and father of mankind. Without them we'd be nothing." The initials identifying this script are worn and faint, but look like "'03 DE," and given my class listings for 2003 it would likely be Dan Elmowitz. I would like to think his small gesture of reverence for Nature has an effect, as any run in the right direction is also a gesture that does. In running, as they say, the hardest and the most important step is always the first one out the door. Everyone can do it, and it counts.

We strive to be worthy, and as social beings we frame our worthiness in terms of becoming part of something we deem to be of value that is greater than ourselves, such as a sports team, a clan, a country. Why not of Nature, to which we all belong, and especially now as we are ever more cosmopolitan? Can we learn enough to love and want and act to take steps, any step, to keep it? It would unite us all, in everlasting grandeur and beauty.

At the school I attended as a young boy in Maine, self-worth required church religion, being able to wash and iron our Sunday white shirts to get ready for the service, reciting the Lord's Prayer in church and before study hour in the evening, and paying deference to a flag at the convocations before classes in high school. If we had thought about it, we would have been confused. But we were kids searching for certainty to live by. So we didn't ask questions. I felt pressured, especially because I was an outsider. So much seemed abstract, confusing, logic defying. I would not have been lonely and unsettled if we had been taught that Nature is God. *That* I would have understood and would have loved to devote myself to.

Having now passed my eightieth birthday, I'm no longer the runner or the scientist I once was, but I've had most of my dreams come true. Both roles had until recently captured my focus and energies. I'm sorry that I was all too often unable to give more attention to relationships and friends. My new race in the last passage of my life is to learn to love more deeply after a lifetime of having to repress my feelings in order to focus on self-reliance and urgent tasks, therefore missing the fullness of life in my family and friends.

There are still many unknowns along the road ahead before the finish line. But what will serve me well from the past is my perseverance and discipline and applying them to whatever may come. Some of my passions will continue: my love of birds, insects, trees . . . and all the new realms that are dawning. I'll learn new skills to communicate with my friends and admirers. I will continue to love the wilderness for its freedom to transform and begin to live what has been unconscious. It will be a metamorphosis from what I was, the awakening of the too long dormant seeds within, and the hope of passing some on, as so much was passed on to me.

I'm looking back also to all my eight professors who inspired me. There were six from the University of Maine and two from UCLA, all names I remember fondly. All are now deceased. I am no longer a professor and heading toward the beyond. When I reach the finish of my longest run, I would not want to be confined in a box, not on the ground but surrounded by it. I'd like it to be a party in the woods, one like any at the end of an ultramarathon, with free beers for all to celebrate my send-off back into Nature, back to the starting line where it all began. I'd like the occasion to be a celebration, with rock music from folks using their minds and instruments, like we had around the table with the many names and inscriptions. The soil around me would serve well to plant and grow an American chestnut tree, *Castanea dentata*. All participants would be free to search for a seedling in the neighboring forest, to take home to plant for themselves. Finally, I would think of them knowing I wish them the best while they are running a loop around Webb Lake via Westbrook Road and past the foot of Mount Tumbledown, where Floyd Adams's several words had motivated a foreign kid new to this country to try to become a runner—and hopefully a citizen of the world.

Acknowledgments

RUNNING MAY BE SOLITARY AT TIMES, AS DESCRIBED IN ALAN
Sillitoe's *The Loneliness of the Long-Distance Runner*, but there are
always companions. A life experience of running is entwined
with inspiring and wonderful people, and this book is dedicated
to runners, friends, associates, competitors, and teammates who
have, as has every mile run, left a mark. They are a part of this
book. Running is a communal enterprise in which we cheer for
and empathize with others. I thank the officials who selflessly
give of their time and am grateful for their devotion to running
events. I thank my teammates of two high school cross-country
years and my mentors and early teachers, Floyd Adams, Phil
and Myrtle Potter, and many teachers for their incredible patience with me at the Good Will–Hinckley School, especially
Lefty Gould, Winfred Kelly, Esther Dunham, Phil Towle, and
Donald Price. From the four years with the University of Maine
cross-country, indoor track, and spring varsity track teams I still
carry the faces, cheers, and gestures of their running spirit with
me. The late coaches Bob Colby and Edmund Styrna stand out
in my memory. I thank Max Mische, my now fifty-year running colleague from our ten years of running on UC Berkeley's
Edwards Track, and our mutual friend, mentor, and informal

coach there, Mark Gruby. Max has refreshed my memory of our experiences then, which will never be forgotten.

I owe as much if not more to all those who contributed to the science that has animated and inspired me. I was weaned on the books on environmental and insect physiology by Knut Schmidt-Nielsen and Sir Vincent Wigglesworth. Others are too numerous to mention and are for the most part known to me only by their contributions to the scientific literature. Personally, however, I owe gratitude to my undergraduate and master's degree mentors at the University of Maine, all of whom I still vividly remember for their inspiration, unfailing support, and friendship: Professors James R. Cook, Al Barden, Ken Allen, Ben Speicher, Charles Major, Bill Valleau, Alan Mun, and Frank Roberts, and at UCLA George A. Bartholomew and Franz Engelmann.

Of more recent vintage, I thank the late Bill Gayton for his devotion to the Southern Maine Rowdies Track Club, of which I was not an official but I believe an honorary member, and I carry that honor proudly. Race director Gayton was a friend, helper, and fighter for runners' rights. I miss his cheer and his gumption. Thanks to my Rowdies teammate Darren Billings for coming up with the bright idea of my trying to achieve a US record on the track, convincing me that it was possible, and then getting me there, and Charles F. Sewall for staying up all night to help keep me hydrated and nourished on the track and providing rides to Boston and to various races; Lynn Jennings, one of the most accomplished middle-distance runners of our time, for hanging out and running with me for seven wonderful years; Jason Mazurowski for a tip that changed my running direction, and Donne Sinderson for her karma to get me up and running for my first ultra after a more than thirty-year hiatus, her remembrance of our celebration of it, and her invaluable help as typist. I thank Edward O. Wilson for arranging and supporting my sabbatical stay at Harvard, and his encouragement to get me onto the marathon path. I am grateful for the gift of his book *The Future of Life*, which he generously inscribed with a sketch of an ant and "For Bernd, with affection and admiration."

Many others from the distant past and into the present to whom I'm grateful for their interest and who in one way or another influenced me in my running and my science include Jack Fultz, Ray Krolewicz, Rick Krause, Jeff Fleitz, Matt Laye, John Scibetta, Benjamin Keller, Aaron Baggish, David Huish, and Charles Sawyer, and Nancy Bowker for her grit and inspirations.

Many thanks and deep gratitude to my agent, Sandra Dijkstra; my editor, Gabriella Doob; and the staff at HarperCollins for their generous support, encouragement, and patience.

REFERENCES

Billings, D. "Aerobic Efficiency in Ultrarunners." *UltraRunning,* November 1984, 24–25.

Cobb, M. *Life's Greatest Secret: The Race to Crack the Genetic Code.* London: Profile Books, 2015.

Cook, J. R., and B. Heinrich. "Glucose vs. Acetate Metabolism in *Euglena.*" *Journal of Protozoology* 12, no. 4 (1965): 581–84.

Costill, D. L. "A Scientific Approach to Distance Running." *Track and Field News,* 1979.

DeCoursey, P. J. "Effect of Light on the Circadian Activity Rhythms of the Flying Squirrel, *Glaucomys volans.*" *Zeitschrift für Vergleichende Physiologie* 44 (1961): 331–54.

Dunlap, J. C. "Molecular Bases for Circadian Clocks." *Cell* 96, no. 2 (January 22, 1999): 271–90.

Gwinner, E. "Photoperiodic Synchronization of Circannual Rhythms in the European Starling (*Sturnus vulgaris*)." *Naturwissenschaften* 64 (1977): 44–45.

Gwinner, E., and J. Dittami. "Pineal Influences on Circannual Cycles in European Starlings: Effects Through the Circadian System?" In *Vertebrate Circadian Systems: Structure and Physiology,* edited by J. Aschoff, S. Daan, and G. A. Groos, 276–84. Berlin: Springer-Verlag, 1982.

Hayes, G. L. T., et al. "Male Semelparity and Multiple Paternity in an Arid-Zone Dasyurid." *Journal of Zoology* 308, no. 4 (April 21, 2019): 266–73.

Heinrich, B. "Bee Flowers: A Hypothesis on Flower Variety and Blooming Times." *Evolution* 29, no. 2 (June 1975): 325–34.

———. "Energetics of Honeybee Swarm Thermoregulation." *Science* 212, no. 4494 (May 1981): 565–66.

———. "Energetics of Pollination." *Annual Review of Ecology and Systematics* 6 (November 1975): 139–70.

———. "The Exercise Physiology of the Bumblebee." *American Scientist* 65, no. 4 (July–August 1977): 455–65.

———. "The Foraging Specializations of Individual Bumblebees." *Ecological Monographs* 46, no. 2 (Spring 1976): 105–28.

———. "Heat Exchange in Relation to Blood Flow Between Thorax and Abdomen in Bumblebees." *Journal of Experimental Biology* 64 (1976): 561–85.

———. "Nervous Control of the Heart During Thoracic Temperature Regulation in a Sphinx Moth." *Science* 169, no. 3945 (August 7, 1970): 606–7.

———. "Pacing: The Lesson of the Frogs." *UltraRunning*, July–August 1987, 32–33.

———. *Racing the Antelope: What Animals Can Teach Us About Running and Life.* New York: Ecco, 2001.

———. *The Snoring Bird: My Family's Journey Through a Century of Biology.* New York: Ecco, 2007.

———. "Thermoregulation in Bumblebees: II. Energetics of Warm-up and Free Flight." *Journal of Comparative Physiology* 96 (June 1975): 155–66.

———. "Thermoregulation in Endothermic Insects." *Science* 185, no. 4153 (August 30, 1974): 747–56.

———. "Thoracic Temperature Stabilization by Blood Circulation in a Free-Flying Moth." *Science* 168, no. 3931 (May 1, 1970): 580–82.

———. "Weasels in Farmington." *Maine Field Naturalist* 17 (1961): 24–25.

———. "Why Have Some Animals Evolved to Regulate a High Body Temperature?" *American Naturalist* 111, no. 980 (July–August 1977): 623–40.

———. *Why We Run: A Natural History.* New York: Ecco, 2001.

Heinrich, B., and G. A. Bartholomew. "Roles of Endothermy and Size in Inter- and Intraspecific Competition for Elephant Dung in an African Dung Beetle, *Scarabaeus laevistriatus.*" *Physiological Zoology* 52, no. 4 (October 1979): 484–96.

Heinrich, B., and J. R. Cook. "Studies on the Respiratory Physiology of *Euglena gracilis* Cultured on Acetate or Glucose." *Journal of Protozoology* 14, no. 4 (November 1967): 548–53.

Heinrich, B., and C. Pantle. "Thermoregulation in Small Flies (*Syrphus* sp.): Basking and Shivering." *Journal of Experimental Biology* 62 (1975): 599–610.

Jordan, W. "The Bee Complex." *Science* 5 (May 1984): 58–65.

Kammer, A. E., and B. Heinrich. "Metabolic Rates Related to Muscle Activity in Bumblebees." *Journal of Experimental Biology* 61, no. 1 (August 1974): 219–27.

Kessel, E. L. "The Mating Activities of Balloon Flies." *Systematic Zoology* 4, no. 3 (September 1955): 97–104.

Krause, R. *One Hundred Years of Maine Running* (self-pub., 1995).

McKenzie, P. "When Do Ultrarunners Stop Running Ultras?" *UltraRunning* (April 1992): 31.

Miller, B. F., et al. "Participation in a 1,000-Mile Race Increases the Oxidation of Carbohydrate in Alaskan Sled Dogs." *Journal of Applied Physiology* 118 (June 2015): 1502–9.

Noakes, T. *The Lore of Running.* Cape Town: Oxford University Press Southern Africa, 1985.

Parker, J. L., Jr. *Once a Runner.* New York: Cedarwinds, 1978.

Pérez-Rodríguez, L., et al. "Vitamin E Supplementation—But Not Induced Oxidative Stress—Influences Telomere Dynamics During Early Development in Wild Passerines." *Frontiers in Ecology and Evolution* 7:173 (May 21, 2019).

Renner, M. "Über ein weiteres Versetzungsexperiment zur Analyse des Zeitsinnes und der Sonnenorientierung der Honigbiene." *Zeitschrift für Vergleichende Physiologie* 42 (September 1959): 449–83.

Riegel, P. "The Aging Slowdown." *UltraRunning,* December 1984, 30.

Sillitoe, A. *The Loneliness of the Long-Distance Runner.* New York: Alfred A. Knopf, 1959.

Svensson, P. *The Book of Eels*. New York: Ecco, 2020.

Taigen, T. L., and K. D. Wells. "Energetics of Vocalization by an Anuran Amphibian (*Hyla versicolor*)." *Journal of Comparative Physiology B* 155 (1985): 163–70.

Thomas, E. M. *The Old Way: A Story of the First People*. New York: Sarah Crichton Books, 2006.

Travis, J. "Chilled Brains." *Science News* 152 (1997): 364–65.

Van der Post, L. *The Lost World of the Kalahari*. Harmondsworth, UK: Hogarth Press, 1958.

Von Frisch, K. *Bees: Their Vision, Chemical Senses, and Language*. Ithaca, NY: Cornell University Press, 1950.

Ybarrondo, B. A., and B. Heinrich. "Thermoregulation and Response to Competition in the African Dung Ball-Rolling Beetle *Kheper nigroaeneus* (Coleoptera: Scarabaeidae)." *Physiological Zoology* 69 (1996): 35–48.

Young, M. W. "The Tick-Tock of the Biological Clock." *Scientific American* 282, no. 3 (March 2000): 64–71.